Medical IELTS

A workbook for international doctors and PLAB candidates

Edited by

David Sales FRCGP

General Practitioner, West Sussex
Deputy Convenor, MRCGP (UK) Examination
International Development Adviser, MRCGP [International]
Member, GMC PLAB Part 1 Panel

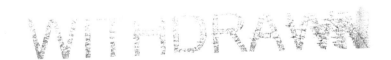

Radcliffe Publishing
Oxford • San Francisco

Radcliffe Publishing Ltd
18 Marcham Road
Abingdon
Oxon OX14 1AA
United Kingdom

www.radcliffe-oxford.com
Electronic catalogue and worldwide online ordering facility.

British Library Cataloguing in Publication Data

A catalogue record for this book is available from the British Library.

ISBN 1 85775 862 5

Radcliffe Publishing Ltd would like to acknowledge the help and co-operation of Bloomsbury plc
in authorising the inclusion of *IELTS Examination: a workbook for students* by Rawdon Wyatt as
Part Two of this book.

Typeset by Anne Joshua & Associates, Oxford
Printed and bound by TJ International Ltd, Padstow, Cornwall

Contents

Part Two

General vocabulary

Topic specific vocabulary

Introduction

This book is aimed primarily to help international medical graduates (IMG) and other international healthcare workers who wish to work in the British National Health Service (NHS) and will be especially helpful for those doctors who may be studying for the International English Language Testing System (IELTS) and subsequently the General Medical Council (GMC) Professional Linguistic Assessment Board (PLAB) Part 2 examination.

Language has been divided into three levels: the technical, the ordinary, and slang or idiom (demotic).[1]

When doctors communicate with each other it is perfectly appropriate to use technical language but, in order to facilitate communication in medical consultations with patients, technical language may be reframed using ordinary language, colloquial language or even idiom or slang. Fluency in idiom or slang is normally acquired through informal contacts and networks rather than through educational means, but such language can be very important in medical communication.[2]

Clearly it is helpful for doctors to be able to explain some of the common and complex medical terms with simple words that are in everyday use by patients and this book offers a means of acquiring proficiency in the use of such words.

On occasion, doctors may resort to idiom or slang, especially in dealing with subjects that may be considered embarrassing, either to the patient or to the doctor, such as toilet functions.

Similarly, patients will avoid using some emotive words such as **cancer**, which may be mentioned as concern about *something serious*, *a growth* or *the big C*, and some doctors are reluctant to use the word **cancer** and use words such as **tumour**, **malignancy** or *growth* instead.

The (mis)use of jargon by the general public is common to all branches of medicine, so that, for example, a headache may be *bad*, an *acute* headache even worse and a *chronic* headache practically unbearable,[3] whereas doctors would use the terms **acute** or **chronic** to describe the duration of symptoms. Should the pain be perceived as being even worse it may be stated (dramatically) that *it's killing me*.

There are some generic terms that patients may use to describe their symptoms, especially when they feel that they are *going down with something* and feel **general malaise** (*non-specifically ill*), which may be described as feeling *under the weather, below par, out of sorts, off colour* or *(really) poorly* or *(really) rotten* or *(really) rough*.

Adjectives are used by patients to denote **severity** of their symptoms so that, for example, a *touch of flu* is a mild bout which typically is a **coryza** (*head cold*). Similarly, a **febrile** or **pyrexial** patient may describe having a *fever* or a *temperature*, but this may be embellished as a *raging temperature* if a patient feels particularly hot, in which case they may maintain that they're *burning up*.

How to use the book

Part One

Part One describes the technical terms that may be used by doctors in **bold**, the ordinary or slang words that may be used by patients in *italic*, and technical words that may be used by both doctors and patients in ***bold italic***. Statements and questions which relate to communication by doctors, especially those that might be used by an IMG, are shown in (parentheses) and those that are suggested for use in UK medical practice are shown in (***bold parentheses***).

Chapters include general advice on history taking and appropriate communication during a physical examination, followed by specific advice using a body system-based approach. Each chapter not only focuses on key words that may be used by both patients and doctors, but also includes a section on communication to facilitate both clinical practice and performance in examinations, such as the PLAB Part 2.

In order to avoid unnecessary duplication some systems are described in more detail than others, but the same principles apply in each case.

Part Two

Part Two has been written for students who are planning to sit either the general training or the academic modules of the IELTS exam. It covers some of the main vocabulary points that you will need for, or come across in, the listening, reading, writing and speaking sections of the exam.

We hope that you find the modules useful and that the vocabulary you acquire will help you to achieve the grade you want in the IELTS.

Good luck!

Structure

Each vocabulary area is presented in the form of a self-contained module with task-based activities which present each vocabulary item in a real context.

- Modules 1–33 focus on general vocabulary items which can be used in all aspects of your English. Some of these are relevant to specific tasks in the IELTS exam (for example, describing how something works, writing a letter or describing a table).

- Modules 34–54 focus on topic-specific vocabulary areas which may be required in the exam (for example, education, business and industry or global problems). Each module consists of three tasks: the first two present vocabulary items in context, and the third gives you the opportunity to review the vocabulary in the form of a gap-fill exercise.

You should not go through the modules mechanically. It is better to choose areas that you are unfamiliar with, or areas that you feel are of specific interest or importance to you.

Vocabulary record sheet

Remember that you should keep a record of new words and expressions that you learn, and review these from time to time so that they become an active part of your vocabulary. There is a vocabulary record sheet at the back of the book which you can photocopy as many times as you like and use to build up your own personal vocabulary bank.

Extending your vocabulary

Also remember that there are other methods of acquiring new vocabulary. For example, you should read as much as possible from a different variety of authentic reading materials (books, newspapers, magazines, etc).

Using an English dictionary

To help you learn English, you should use an English dictionary that can clearly define words, provide information about grammar and give sample sentences to show how words are used in context. You can use any good learner's English dictionary with this book, but it has been written using the material in the *Easier English Dictionary for Students* (2003) by Kathy Rooney (ed.) (ISBN 074756 624 0), published by Peter Collin Publishing, www.petercollin.com.

International English Language Testing System (IELTS)

This book has been written to help you improve your vocabulary when working towards the International English Language Testing System (IELTS) examination. The IELTS English examination is administered by the university of Cambridge Local Examinations Syndicate, The British Council and IDP Education Australia. For further information, please visit www.ucles.org.uk.

Notes

1 Austin JL (1955) *How to Do Things with Words*. Clarendon Press, Oxford.
2 Ali N (2003) *British Journal of General Practice*. **53**: 514–15.
3 Rule A (2003) Shocking language. *BMJ*. **327**: 422.

Part One

1 Communication with patients: general points

Greeting and introduction (*see also* Module 31: Useful interview expressions and Module 40: Healthcare)

When introducing oneself, the statement **Hello/good morning/how do you do? My name is Dr . . . . I'm the SHO from the . . . . department'** is fine for most occasions.

It is useful to know how best to address a patient and in general it is preferable to err on the side of formality and address patients by their **style** and **surname** (*second name*), but sometimes clarification is justified and in such cases questions asked by an IMG might include:

- 'How may I address you?'

- 'How may I call you?'

But **'Is it alright (OK) to call (address) you by your first name?'** is fine, when appropriate.

Thereafter it is vital for any medical consultation to start well and a number of opening questions might be asked by an IMG, including:

- 'How are you doing today/this morning?'

- 'How is your day?'

- 'How are you feeling today?'

- 'How are you?'

However, these questions are generally unsatisfactory in a medical consultation as the patient usually has some complaint.

So . . . it is preferable to ask a question such as follows below:

Presenting problem and addressing patients' concerns

In a hospital outpatient department the reason for a patient's attendance may be explicitly (*openly*) obvious, but in a number of other settings the reason for a patient attending may be less clear and so it is vital to discover the reason for attendance by asking questions such as:

- **'How can I help you?'** or

- **'How would you like me to help you?'**

either of which will suffice in the majority of instances, followed up when appropriate by a question to encourage the patient's contribution such as: **'Could you tell me more about your problem/condition/illness?'**

Thereafter, it is important that the doctor obtains sufficient information to exclude any serious pathology by taking a formal and systematic or appropriately focused medical history as described in the following chapters.

Sometimes it's important to frame the questions, and good examples that might be used by an IMG include:

- 'Sorry to have to ask you these questions.'

- 'I understand that you have a problem of a sensitive/personal nature.'

- 'Is it alright/OK to ask you some personal questions?' or

- 'I am sorry, but I hope that you understand that I have to ask these questions.'

Having heard the patient's story, unless it is already totally obvious, it is usually helpful to enquire what they think their problem might be and an IMG might proceed with a variety of questions to address the patient's concerns, including:

- 'May I/can I know/address your concerns/fears?'

- 'May I know exactly what is your concern/what you are concerned about?'

- 'What is your complaint?'

- 'Which is your problem?'

- 'Have you any complaints to tell me?'

- 'Would you please tell me why you're worried?'

- 'What are your fears?'

- 'You are having a few apprehensions.'

In general, a better response is elicited if the doctor can integrate the patient's concern with their presenting symptom with a question style such as **'Is it the . . . . (chest pain etc) that you are worried about or what may be causing it?'**

Pain

When patients present with **pain**, questions that an IMG might ask include:

- 'Is there any pain in your body?
- 'Where is it paining you?'

But **'Do you have any pain?'** works just as well and could be followed up with appropriate questions to discover the site, character, aggravating and relieving factors, associations and radiation.

Patients and doctors may use adjectives (*see* also Introduction) to describe pain in different ways, so, for example, the word **lancinating** wouldn't be used by patients, who may describe such pain as *sharp* or *shooting*; or **boring** (pain) which they might understand as being a *dull pain like toothache*.

Radiation is another word that has a specific medical meaning but patients may sometimes use the term to describe *diffuse* or *poorly localised* pain.

2 History taking

Occupations (*jobs*) and certificates (*sick notes*) (*see also* Module 36: Work and Module 37: Money and finance)

It is invariably helpful to enquire how a medical problem affects a patient's daily life/ lifestyle or work.

Communication

Examples of questions that might be asked by an IMG include:

- 'In which occupation are you?'

- 'What work are you doing?'

The questions **'What is your job/occupation/work?'** or **'What do you do for a living?'** would normally elicit a straightforward response, but occasionally may require further clarification, as the responses may include being:

- *in retail:* including a variety of occupations such as being a **shop assistant**;

- *in marketing:* including any aspect of **sales**;

- *in IT:* **(information technology)** which may include computer programming or operating;

- *in management:* at any level;

- *in the city:* which may include a variety of financial or business occupations such as being an **insurance broker**;

- *in HR:* **(human resources)**;

- *a civil servant:* working for the central government as opposed to *local government*;

- *a carer:* who would be involved in looking after a person with a particular need for care.

Specific occupations may be volunteered such a being a *joiner* or *chippy* **(carpenter)**, *copper* or *the Old Bill* (***policeman***) and there are a number of other terms that are used by professions when referring to each other that are less likely to be volunteered in the medical context.

Earning **money** (*dosh, bread*) may be referred to as *being the breadwinner* or *paying the rent*.

People may talk of *burning the candle at both ends* when they are getting up early to go to work/study and then staying up late.

Redundancy would be referred to as being *sacked* and when workers take retirement they may receive a *golden handshake* **(lump sum)** followed by a pension, after which time they are referred to as ***pensioners***.

Being unemployed may be referred to as being *on the dole* (claiming unemployment benefits) as opposed to being *on the sick* (incapable of work due to health reasons).

A **medical certificate** for **Department of Social Security (DSS)** benefits is known as a *sick note* or *sickness certificate* or, in Scotland, a *line*.

Cigarettes (*smoking*)

Communication

Questions that might be asked by an IMG include:

- 'Do you have a habit of smoking?'
- 'Since when have you been smoking?'
- 'From how long have you been smoking?'
- 'You were smoking since . . .?'

But **'Do you smoke?'** is just as effective and can be followed up by:

- **'How long have you been smoking for?'**
- **'How many packs a day?'**

Smoking

Some patients smoke roll-ups (*rollies*), which involves buying tobacco sold in pouches weighing multiples of 12.5g and cigarette papers, often known by the brand name *Rizla*.

Pipe-smoking and cigar-smoking are less prevalent.

If patients consider that they are heavy smokers then they may report that they *smoke like a chimney*.

Alcohol (*booze*)

Patients have grown to accept that being questioned about their alcohol consumption by doctors is part of routine history taking or health promotion, although some patients remain **teetotal** (abstain from drinking).

Communication

A number of questions might be used by an IMG to discuss alcohol consumption including:

- 'Is it alright to talk about your alcohol consumption?'
- 'Do you drink alcohol?'

- 'Do you take alcohol at all?'

- 'Do you take any alcohol/drinks?'

- 'Do you take drinks?'

- 'What is the amount of (whisky) that you take?'

- 'What is your usual routine?'

- 'Are you in the habit of taking alcohol?'

- 'What is the maximum that you drink every day?'

- 'Since when have you been drinking?'

But the more standard question that would be used in UK medical practice is:

- **'How many (alcoholic) drinks do you have a day/week?'** or

- **'What is your typical (daily/weekly) alcohol consumption?'**

which may generate responses such as 'Two pints a day and a glass of wine with meals'. However, sometimes the initial question needs to be followed up with a question such as:

- **'What do you normally drink?'**

Many patients are aware of the concept of a unit of alcohol but it is as well to check their understanding (and honesty) before asking:

- **'How many units of alcohol/drinks do you drink per day/week?'**

Sometimes the response suggests no cause for concern and it's sensible to acknowledge this with a reassuring statement such as might be used by an IMG including:

- 'You are normal with that'.

But **'That's fine'** would suffice.
  The patient's response may require some health promotion advice such as:

- **'Have you ever felt that you should cut down on your drinking?'**

rather than the alternatives that are sometimes used, such as:

- 'Do you feel that you are too much dependent on it?'

or advice which may be received negatively such as:

- 'You should cut down on that.'

The more gentle approach of suggesting that the patient might consider the health benefits of having some regular ***dry*** **(abstinent)** days is often more successful.

Drinking – general information

'Fancy a beer/few beers?' has become a generic invitation for having a drink. Down the *pub* **(public house)** customers drink *bitter* **(beer)** or lager in *pints* or sometimes *halves* **(half-pints)** and these are served in a variety of glasses, some with handles and some without, known as *jugs* or *jars*. They also serve other drinks such as **spirits** (*the hard stuff*), including **whisky**, which are served as single *shots* **(single measure)**, sometimes known as a *small Scotch* (whisky), or *doubles* **(double measure)**, sometimes known as a *large measure*.

Aperitifs are fortified wines, such as **sherry**, that are often drunk before meals, in glasses known as a *schooners*. **Wine**, red or white, would typically be consumed with a meal in a restaurant and is measured in glasses known as *goblets* and sparkling wine such as **champagne** in glasses known as *flutes*. Typically, a bottle of wine will contain about nine units of alcohol, but this varies depending on the type and the wines are often described by either their grape type, such as *Shiraz* or *Chardonnay*, or region of origin, such as *New World*.

Some bars sell **cocktails** that have unlikely names such as *Bloody Mary* – which is a mixture of tomato juice and vodka. Other combinations of drinks might include a **spirit**, such as gin, to which is added a **mixer** such as **tonic water**. **Mineral** or **spring water** is **bottled water**, which is widely available although it is perfectly acceptable to drink **tap water.**

At home people may drink cans of beer bought in an **off-licence** (liquor store) or supermarket. They may be sold as a *six-pack* (packet of six) and the Australian fashion of calling these *tinnies* is catching on. Bottled beer is sometimes sold in short, dumpy bottles known as *stubbies* on account of their appearance, or *twisties* on account of the unscrewing top. Younger drinkers are keen on bottles of carbonated alcoholic drinks, known as ***alcopops***, which are often known by their brand names such as *Breezer*.

At home many alcoholic beverages are consumed and people talk about having a *glass* of any sort of alcohol, which maybe described as *stiff* (a stiff drink), *hefty* (measure) or *large* (glass).

Alcohol sometimes is referred to in slang as *booze, sauce, pop* or *grog*, but most patients wouldn't initiate these terms during a medical consultation. However, some patients will use terms such as having a *sniff*, meaning having a quick drink, while they may describe embarking on a **binge** as going on a *session* or *bender*. When describing the effects of alcohol, patients may describe getting *merry, tipsy, pissed, smashed, trolleyed, trashed, hammered* or *rat-arsed*. It's rare that patients admit to having an *eye opener* or *the hair of a dog*, when they take a drink first thing in the morning.

If this is the case then it suggests that a patient has an **alcohol dependence problem** and such patients may develop other symptoms such as ***DTs*** **(delirium tremens)** and need admitting to be *dried out* **(alcoholic detoxification)**. If successful, they remain *dry* or *on the wagon* **(abstinent)**.

Recreational drugs (*drugs*)

Communication

Sometimes patients may present requesting treatment for substance misuse or dependence and on other occasions it's appropriate to enquire about the non-medical use of drugs using a closed question such as: 'Do you take any recreational drugs?'

Phrases that might be used by an IMG include:

- 'I'd like to congratulate you on asking for help.'
- 'Are you motivated to leave the drug?'

But **'Have you made up your mind to stop/quit?'** or **'Have you thought about quitting?'** are probably preferable. *See also* Module 14: Stopping something.

When taking a drug history it's helpful to know some of the language used by drug-users in order to avoid the pitfalls associated with the too-formal questioning that might sometimes be used by an IMG such as:

- 'How do you apply it?'
- 'What is the method that you take it?'
- 'Are you taking it through veins?'
- 'Do you use a solid needle?'

'Are you injecting?' is simpler and would be understood by the majority of users.

'We will be refraining you from doing this' is a cumbersome way of explaining the principles encompassed by **'We will be referring you for *detox* (detoxification) or *rehab* (rehabilitation) and/or a self-help group.'**

'How do you finance your habit?' will help identify those regular users who may resort to petty crime, such as shoplifting, to fund their habit, which may enable questions such as:

- **'Have you ever been in trouble with the law?'**

To which they may respond that they have *been in trouble with/nicked/busted/pulled* **(arrested)** *by Dibble/the Old Bill/the law* **(the police)**.

- **'Have you ever been imprisoned or in jail?'**

If so, patients may respond by saying that they have *served time*, been *inside*, *banged up* or *in the clink*, *done Porridge* or *done bird*. *See also* Module 42: Crime and the law.

Specific drugs

Cannabis (*marihuana, hashish, pot, blow, ganga, grass, resin, dope, dagga, weed* and many more) typically is smoked to get *stoned* in a *bong* **(pipe)** or *joint* (***reefer***) which is rolled by the smoker, often with tobacco in cigarette papers known as *skins* or *Rizlas*, one of the more popular brands, and inserting a self-made tip known as a *roach*.

Heroin (*H, horse*): Users initially seek a *kick* (**excitement**) from their *junk* (**drug**) but may become ***hooked*** (**addicted**) as a ***junkie*** (**heroin addict**) and may *score* (**buy**) their *wrap/fix/gear* from a *connection/dealer/pusher/peddler* (**supplier**) and use (and re-use or share) *works/tools/kit* (**syringe and needles**) or *spikes/nails/bangers* (**needles**) to *shoot/ jab/jack up/jolt/crank up/main-line* (**inject**) the drug, often withdrawing a *splash* (**spurt of blood**) before *flushing* (**injecting back into the vein**). **Needle exchange** schemes encourage the use of *clean* rather than the re-use of *dirty works*. *Chasing the dragon* refers to the practice of heating heroin placed on foil over a flame and **inhaling (smoking) the fumes**.

Cold turkey is used to describe specifically part of the rapid withdrawal from heroin (although the term is sometimes applied to the rapid withdrawal from any drug) and relates to the hair on the skin standing up and the skin itself feeling cold, appearing as ***goose-pimples***.

Cocaine (*coke, charlie, dust, smack, rocks, crack*): A line of coke may be *cut* or *chalked* and is usually *snorted* (**inhaled**) but a user will *crack rocks* and *crack* (**cocaine**) typically is smoked.

Glossary of other main recreational drugs

- **Amfetamines** (amphetamines): *Speed* or *whizz*.

- ***Brown sugar***: Partially refined heroin.

- ***Ecstasy*** (**MDMA**): *E, XTC, smilers, diamonds*; popular in the clubbing scene.

- ***LSD***: *Acid* taken by an *acid head* (**regular user**). A *bad trip* is a *bummer* (**bad/ unpleasant experience**) which may cause the taker to *freak out*.

- ***Magic mushrooms*** (**Liberty Cap**): contain the **hallucinogenic** (*mind-altering*) agent psilocibin. They grow in parks and on golf courses, particularly in the autumn.

- **Ketamine** (*Special K*).

- **Hypnotics** (*sleepers*): such as temazepam may be referred to as *jellies* (after the capsules) or *mazzies*; **mogadon** as *moggies*; **chloral hydrate** as *knock-out drops*.

- **Volatile substances** (inhalation of): ***Glue-sniffing*** including other **volatile sub-stances** such as **butane**, often **inhaled from a bag**.

Diet and nutrition (*food*) (*see also* Module 45: Food and diet)

Obesity (*being fat, a bit overweight or flabby* or *carrying too much*) and unhealthy eating is rife in the UK. Some patients talk of fighting the **middle-age spread**, but many patients of all ages are on self-imposed weight-reducing diets which they may describe as *fighting the flab* and which they may refer to by name such as the (*Dr*) *Atkins diet*.

Communication

A **dietary history** is often relevant for a variety of medical conditions. Examples of good open questions that might be used by an IMG include:

- 'Tell me about your diet.'

- 'What are your eating habits?'

- 'What type of food do you eat/normally take?'

But such questions are likely to generate an imprecise response. It is often necessary to clarify the focus of the dietary enquiry such as:

- **'How many portions of fresh fruit/vegetables do you have a day?'**

- **'Do you have a low fat/low salt/low sugar/high fibre diet?'** as appropriate

- **'Do you skip (miss) any meals?'**

When discussing a low fat diet, patients may tell you that they drink full-fat (4%), semi-skimmed (2%) or skimmed (1%) milk.

People talk about *convenience foods* these may include *take-away foods* such as *fish and chips, burgers, curry* or *cook-chill ready-meals*, bought from supermarkets such as Marks & Spencer and reheated in a microwave.

Slang words for food include *grub, tucker, nosh* and *trough*, but these are not often used in the medical context.

The term ***anorexia*** would normally be used by patients to mean having no appetite or going off their food, and many would reserve the term *anorexia* for the context of the specific eating disorder **anorexia nervosa**.

Exercise

Communication

Questions that might be asked by an IMG include:

- 'Do you take/make regular exercise?'

- 'Do you do any exercises?'

- 'Do you play any sports?'

Such closed questions may need a follow-up question which asks for more details such as the specific nature, frequency and duration of the activity, such as: **'How much exercise do you take in a typical week?'**

For infirm patients it may be more appropriate to reframe the question:

- 'Can you move around at home/in the house?'

- 'Can you do the shopping?'

Being a *couch potato* is a term that is used to describe inactivity but many patients will describe specific activities such as walking (*going for a stroll* or *rambling*), a round of golf, going to the gym – which may include working out or attending specific classes or activities such as aerobics or Pilates, running (***jogging***) and football (***soccer***).

Other social history

When appropriate it may be helpful to ask relevant details to place the patient's complaint in the following social contexts (*settings*). Questions that might be asked by an IMG include:

- 'Since how long have you been living here?'

But **'How long have you lived here?'** is readily understood by the majority.
   A **homeless** person may say that they *live rough* or *on the streets*.

In terms of assessing the relationship in a family, the questions that might be asked by an IMG include:

- 'Do you maintain links with your family?'

But **'How is your relationship with your family?'** would probably be more effective. *See also* Module 46: Children and the family.

In terms of **hobbies** or **interests** it is sometimes helpful to ask, where appropriate, a question such as might be asked by an IMG:

- 'Do you take an interest in any activities?'

Or: **'What are your interests/hobbies?'**

3 Gastro-intestinal (*digestive*) system

Patients use a number of colloquial terms when describing their bodily functions, none more so than in the gastro-intestinal system.

Heartburn and water-brash or acidity are descriptions for symptoms which may be caused by **gastro-oesophageal reflux disease (GORD)**, although patients tend to refer to their *gullet* rather than their **oesophagus**. Feeling **nauseous** may be referred to as *feeling sick*; **reflux** may be described as *heaving* or *retching* and **vomiting** as *throwing up* or *honking up* or being *unable to keep anything down*. **Dysphagia** (*difficulty swallowing*) typically would be described as *food getting stuck*.

Eructation may be described as *belching, burping* or *repeating*.

Whilst the word **stomach** has a very specific anatomical or medical meaning, patients may use the precise term in a general sense, for example, *stomach-ache* may refer to *general tummy* or *abdominal pain* or occasionally *belly ache*, and *stomach cramp* may mean any colicky abdominal pain. The **umbilicus** may be referred to as the *navel, belly button* or *tummy button*, which is becoming an increasingly popular site for **body piercing**.

The contents of the peritoneal cavity, but especially the **intestines** or **bowels**, are often referred to as *guts* or occasionally *innards*, and dysfunction may be described by patients as *gut-rot* (for diarrhoea), and *worry-gut* or *sick with worry* for *butterflies in the stomach* (caused by **anxiety**). People may describe a particularly bad experience as being *gut-wrenching* and the generic phrase *feeling gutted* when they are very upset.

Sensations such as *feeling liverish* or *having a bilious attack* are used to describe the collection of symptoms associated with **hepatic** (*liver*) or gall-bladder dysfunction. **Hepatitis** would be understood as an *infection and inflammation of the liver* which may cause signs such as **jaundice**, which is often tautologically described as *yellow jaundice*. Some patients complain that they have *liver spots*, which don't seem to have a medical diagnosis.

Euphemisms, such as having a *number two, big job, big toilet, dump, crap* or *shit* may be rife in society when referring to **bowel movements**, but would be considered to be inappropriate by many in medical consultations.

Communication

Questions that might be asked by an IMG include:

- 'What about your motions?'

- 'Tell me about the passing of your stool.'

- 'Do you have any diarrhoea these days?'

Although patients generally understand the more formal questions such as:

- **'Have you had any change in your bowel habit?'**

- 'How often do you open your bowels?'

- 'Are your bowels opened normally/regularly?'

Patients tend not to use the words such as **motions** or **stools** but would not generally use terms such as *turd* in a medical context, although children (and many adults) will use the word *poo* and some occasionally use the scientific term **excrement**. If they are **constipated** they may talk about being *bunged-up* and **diarrhoea** may be described as *being loose, having the runs/trots* or *the collywobbles* and if sudden may be described as *being caught short*.

A stool sample may need some clarification as the generic word **sample** is often interpreted as being a **urine sample** but an explanation as to the purpose of the test, such as **faecal occult blood (FOB)** (*hidden blood in the stool*) will be helpful.

Flatulence would be described as having *gas* or *passing wind*, but patients generally would avoid using terms such as *fart* in medical consultations. The term **offensive** (as in stool) would typically be understood as *smells bad* or *smelly* and most would understand *slime* rather than **mucus**.

A **rectal (per rectum/pr) examination** is understood as *examining the back-passage* (**anus** and/or **rectum**) as opposed to *an internal*, which is reserved for a **vaginal (per vagina) examination**.

When explaining the findings of a pr most patients would understand **haemorrhoids** although they would use the term *piles* and a **fissure** could be explained as a *split*.

People sit on their ***bottom*** or ***seat*** (***buttocks*** or *cheeks*), which may also be referred to as their *bum*.

Most patients would understand the term ***back passage*** for the **anus** and would generally avoid the more vulgar terms (such as *arse*) in the medical context.

Gastro-intestinal pathology (*disease*)

Irritable bowel syndrome would be understood as a *nervous stomach* causing **colicky** (*crampy/griping*) abdominal pain due to ***spasm (contraction)*** of the ***large intestines (bowels)***.

Gastroenteritis is referred to as ***gastric flu***, which, if severe and especially in children, may lead to **dehydration** (*becoming dry due to losing body fluid*). **Coeliac disease** may be described as having *a wheat sensitivity or intolerance* (although many patients would use the term *allergy*), **colitis** as *inflammation of the bowel causing bad diarrhoea*, **dysentery** as *severe diarrhoea due to an infection* and **paralytic ileus** as *loss of intestinal movement*.

A **hernia** (protrusion of the bowel through a weakness in the abdominal wall muscles) is understood as a *rupture*.

A *stitch* is a disabling pain up under the ribs, which occurs on exertion, more frequently in younger patients, probably originating from the diaphragm.

4 Cardio-vascular system (*heart and circulation*)

Patients with heart disease would describe being under the *heart doctor* or *specialist* (**cardiologist**).

Congenital (*born with*) heart lesions

A **ventricular-septal defect (VSD)** (*hole in the heart*) is typically discovered as a **murmur** (*blowing sound caused by turbulence of the blood in the heart*). A **right to left shunt** (*blood flowing the wrong way*), such as in a **Fallot's tetralogy**, will result in **cyanosis** (*a blue baby*) due to lack of oxygen in the blood. A **coarctation of the aorta** (*narrowing of the main artery/blood vessel leaving the heart*) would be detected by **diminished** (*weak*) **femoral pulses** (*rhythmic throbbing of arteries as blood is propelled by the heart beating and felt in the groin*).

Cardio-vascular problems

Shock is one of those words that most doctors would agree is related to having dangerously *low blood pressure* (**hypotension**) but the term is often used by the British public to include *experiencing a psychologically traumatic event*.

Doctors often advise their patients about **risk factors** for **coronary *heart disease***, which may include a **genetic predisposition** (*a risk inherited from/given by parents*) or a **family history** (*runs in the family*) or **modifiable *lifestyle*** factors such as ***smoking***, ***diet***, ***exercise*** or ***stress***.

Hypertension (*raised/high blood pressure*) is often referred to as having *blood pressure*, and is measured using a **sphygmomanometer** (*blood pressure measuring instrument*).

Patients will talk about their *heart missing a beat* rather than **palpitations**, which they may describe as having a *sensation of feeling their heart (ticker) pounding, beating or fluttering in their chest*. The heart sounds are heard on **auscultation** (*act of listening*) using a **stethoscope** (*listening instrument*).

Sometimes patients will tell you that they have a history of a *weak heart*, which may encompass **any cardiac diagnosis**. ***Angina*** is a term that appears to be widely used and understood and may need **investigation** (*tests*) with an **electrocardiograph (ECG)** (*heart tracing*) or **exercise test** on a treadmill and **venepuncture** (*blood tests*) including **lipids/cholesterol/triglycerides** (*types of fat*).

Further tests may include a **coronary angiogram** (*dye test*), which may reveal a **stenosis** (*narrowing*) or **obstruction** (*blockage*) which may need treatment such as an **angioplasty** (*using a balloon to split a narrow artery to make it bigger to improve the blood supply to the heart muscle*), **stent insertion** (*small tube* for the same purpose) or a coronary artery bypass graft (CABG), referred to by many patients as a *triple/quadruple bypass* (as appropriate).

A **myocardial infarct** (*heart attack*) may need to be treated with **thrombolytic** treatment (*clotbusters*).

A **cardiac arrest** (*heart has stopped*) may be treated with **mouth to mouth resuscitation** (*the kiss of life*) and, if need be, by **cardioversion** or **defibrillation** (*shock*) and putting a patient on a **ventilator** (*life-support machine*).

A **deep vein thrombosis** may be referred to by the initials *DVT* or more typically as a *thrombosis* or *blood-clot*, and a **pulmonary embolus** is understood in terms of *a blood clot that has moved to the lung from the leg* (*or other part of body*).

Anticoagulants are referred to as *blood-thinners* and **atrial fibrillation** as an *irregular heart beat*, which may be treated with an **anti-arrhythmic agent** (*drug to steady an irregular heartbeat*) or **radio-frequency ablation** (*electro-zapping*).

A **tachycardia** is can be understood as a *fast heart rate*, **bradycardia** as a *slow heart rate* and conduction defects including **heart block** as *a delay in the passage/transmission of electrical signals through the heart*.

Cardiac (*heart*) failure is explained as *causing a build up of fluid on the chest and/or ankles* (**oedema**) due to any heart disease which reduces the **cardiac output** (*the heart's ability to work as a pump*) and which may be treated by drugs including **diuretics** (*water pills*).

Peripheral vascular disease can be explained as *furring up* or *narrowing* of the arteries and specific conditions such as **Raynaud's disease** as a *circulation disorder* caused by **vasospasm** (*contraction/spasm [of the blood vessel]*), for which they may be prescribed **vasodilators** (*drugs that dilate blood vessels*), which may cause a side effect such as **orthostatic hypotension** (*temporary drop in blood pressure on standing*).

Restless legs are characterised by symptoms such as feelings of *burning*, *tickling* or *crawling* pain and a *desire to move the limbs* (**akathisia**).

An **aneurysm** would be understood as a *swelling in an artery due to a weakness in the wall* which, if left untreated, may run the risk of a subsequent **rupture** (*leak/burst*).

5 Psychiatry (*nervous disorders*)

A **psychiatrist** may be referred to as *shrink* or a *head doctor* by some patients and **psychiatric hospitals** referred to as *the nut-house, the bin, a loony (lunatic) asylum* or *the funny farm*.

Paradoxically, **psychiatric** (rather than neurological) **illnesses** are often referred to generically as *nervous disorders, weak nerves* or *trouble with the nerves*, and the term *nervous breakdown* is used quite extensively and by patients to signify what they refer to as *clinical depression*.

When patients suffer from *nervous problems* they sometimes fear that they are *cracking up, going mad/crazy/round the bend, losing their marbles, having a screw loose* or *losing the plot* (losing touch with reality) or *going doolally*.

Depression

Patients often find it difficult to express their emotions to a doctor and may describe the sensation of *feeling tired all the time* as having *no energy*, being *exhausted* or *knackered*, of having *legs like lead* if they have no energy or having *bags under their eyes* if they think they look tired due to **insomnia** (*difficulty sleeping*). A **depressed mood** may be described as feeling *low, down, down in the dumps, grumpy, moody, blue, fed up* or *browned off*. Some patients will describe having a *heavy* or *broken heart*, especially if they are distressed by unrequited love.

Euthymia technically describes a *normal mood* while **euphoria** is widely interpreted as being *unduly high*.

Communication

A sensitive style of questioning is especially important when discussing emotional issues and the questions that have been used include the encouraging statement 'Feel free to open your heart out', which is very succinct and conveys the message, but in the UK patients are generally floored by this style.

In general, the questions that appear to work well include:

- **'How do you feel in yourself?'**
- **'How do feel about the future?'**
- **'How do you see your life in general?'**
- **'When did you last have a good day?'**
- **'When were you last happy?'**

When assessing the severity of depression, whilst it is a difficult area to discuss, it is very important to assess suicidal ideation, and appropriate questions include:

- **'Have you ever felt that life wasn't worth living?'**
- **'Have you ever thought about harming yourself?'**
- **'Have you thought how you might do it?'**

Suicide: Patients sometimes talk about *doing something stupid* or occasionally about *harming*, *hurting* or *topping* themselves.

Anxiety

Patients talk about feeling *stressed out*, being *highly strung* or *tense*, being unable to *chill* or *chill out* (relax) or being *bad with their nerves*, and many people use the term **neurotic** to mean *a bit of a worrier*.

Treatment of depression and anxiety

Patients will often refer to **antidepressants** as *happy pills* and **anxiolytics** as *something to calm the nerves*. Most forms of **therapy** would be referred to as ***counselling*** and **electro convulsive therapy (ECT)** as *shock treatment*.

Psychosis

Often this is brought to the attention of the medical profession by a third party and such patients may be described as displaying *unusual behaviour*, which may include being *unduly suspicious* (**paranoid**), *unduly care-free* (**disinhibited**), being *overactive* or a bit *hyper* (meaning **hypomanic**). *Manic depression* has crept into general use for **bipolar affective disorder**.

Derogatory terms for patients with serious psychiatric morbidity include *bonce job*, *head case* or *basket case*.

The term **schizophrenia** appears to be interpreted in the UK as being a bit of a *Jekyll and Hyde*, meaning that an individual has a *split personality* rather than the strict medical diagnosis comprising **first rank symptoms** such as **hallucinations** (*seeing or hearing things*).

6 Neurological system

A **neurosurgeon** is referred to as a *brain surgeon*.

In children **convulsions** are often associated with a febrile illness **(febrile convulsions)** but if **seizures** *(fits)* are recurrent or prolonged it is appropriate to refer for investigation of possible **epilepsy**.

Following a head injury a patient may have ***concussion*** if they have **lost consciousness** *(been knocked out)*.

A *funny turn*, occasionally abbreviated to *turn*, or *coming over queer* are used to describe a number of symptoms including ***blackouts*** **(transient loss of consciousness)**, which may be caused by **vertebro-basilar insufficiency (VBI)** (***a drop attack***, explained as *kinking of the blood supply to the balancing centre in the brain*) or a **transient ischaemic attack (TIA)** *(mini stroke* or *warning)* and may lead to the patient ***going off their legs*** or to a more specific presentation such as **amaurosis fugax** *(curtain coming across the field of vision)*.

Such patients may describe feeling *light-headed, woozy, swimmy, giddy* or *dizzy*, by which they may mean that their *head was spinning*. **True rotational vertigo** has a specific medical interpretation but some patients reserve its use specifically for a sensation that relates to their *discomfort on being at a great height*.

If a patient has had a TIA they may complain of **paraesthesiae** *(pins and needles)* and when investigated may have a CT or MRI scan *(brain scan)*. A **cerebro-vascular accident (CVA)** or ***stroke*** may present with a **hemiplegia** *(weakness of one side)* and **dysphasia** *(difficulty with speech)*.

Movement disorders may present with a ***tremor*** *(shaking)*, **fasciculation** *(twitching)* or **myoclonus** *(jerky movements)*. **Flaccidity** would be understood as being *limp*, wherever the term is used, and **rigidity** as *stiffness*.

Parkinson's disease may present with **bradykinesia** *(slow movements)*, **cog-wheel or lead-pipe rigidity** and a **pill-rolling tremor**.

Patients may present with an **insidious** *(subtle and gradual)* onset of rather vague symptoms such as **asthenia** *(weakness)* and may worry about having ***ME*** **(myalgic encephalomyelitis)**, which is usually referred to by doctors as **chronic fatigue syndrome**. **Atypical** *(unusual)* **presentations** of many neurological conditions are common, such as **multiple sclerosis (*MS*)**.

When patients present with **amnesia** they may describe *becoming forgetful* or *losing their memory*.

7 Ear, nose and throat (ENT) system

Patients sometimes have a **health belief** that leads them to believe that they catch a *chill* from getting cold, but viral upper respiratory tract infections (URTIs) especially a **coryza** (*common head cold*) are common, and patients present with **rhinitis** (*a runny nose*), **nasal obstruction/congestion** (*being bunged up, having a blocked nose*) and/or a **nasal discharge** (*snuffles* or *snotty nose*).

Catarrh is often mentioned and if infected may be described by its colour so that a **muco-purulent discharge** will be *green catarrh*. Sometimes patients will tell you about their *spit*, which may mean **saliva**, **phlegm** or **sputum**, and they may feel that it comes up from their chest rather than being related to post-nasal **discharge** (*drip*).

Inflammation is understood as *swelling*. *Infections* (*germs*) can be explained using the generic term **micro-organisms** (*bugs*) and many patients understand that bacterial germs might respond to antibiotics while viruses don't.

Allergic or **seasonal rhinitis** (*hayfever*) is also common and such patients may have other symptoms including itchy red eyes and may have **conjunctivitis** (*red-eye*).

Epistaxes (*nose bleeds*) are typically expected to be caused by *blood pressure* **(hypertension)** although they rarely are!

Sore throats are common and patients often worry that they may have *tonsillitis* although they usually have **pharyngitis** (*throat infection*) or occasionally **laryngitis** (*infection of the voice box*), which may present with a *frog in the throat* or *gruff voice*. Patients sometimes are confused regarding their oro-pharyngeal anatomy and may think that their **uvula** is their **epiglottis**.

Less commonly patients may present with a *sore (**inflamed**) mouth* (**stomatitis**), a *sore tongue* **(glossitis)**, or *sore gums* **(gingivitis)** in which case they may complain of *bad breath* **(halitosis)**. Patients with *toothache* often attend a doctor with, for example, an **apical abscess** (*gum boil*) and they are better referred to a **dentist** for definitive treatment.

Otalgia (*earache*) is commonly caused by **otitis media** (*middle ear infection*) in children or **otitis externa** (*outer ear infection*) in swimmers, which is why it is known as *swimmer's ear*. The ear is examined by an **auriscope/otoscope** (*small instrument with a light*) to **visualise** (*see*) the **external auditory meatus** (*ear canal*) and **tympanic membrane** (*ear drum*) which may reveal an **effusion** (*fluid in the middle ear*). Occasionally, if this is a **chronic** (*longstanding*) problem a **grommet** (*small tube*) may be **inserted** (*put in*) to **ventilate** (*drain fluid out and allow air in to*) the middle ear.

Happily, as with other many anatomical terms, there is concordance between the patients and medical use of terms like ear, nose and throat, but this does not prevent the use of pet names such as *ear-hole, lug-hole* (ear), *hooter* or *snout* (nose) or *chops, gob* (mouth).

Patients often complain of **deafness** or *popping in their ears* after a head cold due to

eustachian tube dysfunction, which can be explained as *a blockage caused by catarrh in the tube that goes from the back of the throat to the middle ear*.

Occasionally deafness is more permanent and may require referral for an **audiogram** (*hearing test*) for example in **presbyacusis** (*deterioration of hearing with age*).

Less common symptoms include **tinnitus**, which would be described as *ringing*, *buzzing or noises in the ears*; and **globus (hystericus/pharyngeus)**, symptoms which sometimes may be associated with **air hunger** (*feeling of inability to breathe*), although such patients are often investigated for **GORD**.

8 Respiratory (*breathing*) system

Patients with breathing problems will consider that they see *chest specialist* or *chest doctor*.

Patients with **dyspnoea** present complaining of feeling *short of breath, short of puff, out of breath*, being *unable to catch their breath* or occasionally just plain *puffed*.

Following a **coryza** (*head cold*) patients are often concerned that the *infection may be going on their chest* and may talk about *having a chest cold* or *being a bit bronchial*, although they often have **tracheitis** (*infection in their windpipe*).

Children present with a *harsh barking cough* which parents often correctly diagnose as ***croup* (laryngo-tracheo-bronchitis)**, although other causes of **stridor** (*noisy breathing*) such as ***quinsy* (tonsillar abscess)** may need to be excluded; and especially if their child has not been immunised they may be concerned about ***whooping cough* (pertussis)**.

Asthma may be described as being *wheezy* or *tight-chested* or having *bronchial asthma*.

If patients feel that they are **cyanosed** they may describe being a bit *blue round the gills*.

Specific conditions such as **pulmonary fibrosis** could be explained as *thickening and stiffening* (of the lungs).

9 Urogenital and reproductive system

Urology

The process is often discussed in preference to structure, but patients may describe having a *weak bladder* for **any urinary symptoms** but on discussing patients' *waterworks*, patients will talk about ***passing urine***, *having a wee/pee*, *going to the toilet/loo*, or *spending a penny* and will avoid the technical term **micturition**. The term *pissing* would generally not be used in a medical context.

In describing the symptoms of ***cystitis*** patients will complain that they are *going* or *peeing often* (**frequency**), that they have a *burning sensation* (**dysuria**) or more rarely *blood in the urine* (**haematuria**), and are often concerned that they may have a *kidney* (**renal**) infection (**pyelonephritis**), in which case the infection could be explained as ascending (*going up*) the **ureter** (*tube from the kidney to the bladder*). **Loin pain** also raises the possibility of ureteric **colic** (*intense spasm in the ureter*) due to a **calculus** (*stone*).

Children may be presented with **primary nocturnal enuresis** (***bed wetting*** in a child who has never been dry at night) as opposed to **secondary** (*when the child had previously been dry by night*) and it is important to arrange collection of a **mid-stream specimen of urine (mssu)** to exclude a urinary tract infection or diabetes mellitus.

Many middle-aged men develop lower urinary tract symptoms, which may be associated with **benign prostate hypertrophy,** and they understand that the gland gets bigger with age. Such patients will describe: needing to *get up several times at night* (**nocturia**), being *unable to wait* (**urgency**), *difficulty starting to pee* (**hesitancy**), having a *weak flow* or *poor pressure* (**poor stream**), having accidents (**incontinence**).

Sometimes such patients may have an *overactive* or ***irritable bladder*** (**detrusor instability**).

If women suffer from continence problems they may use several of these terms, although they will also talk about *seepage* or *dribbling* or *having accidents*.

Euphemisms are rife with the **anatomy** in this department, which may be referred to generically as *privates*, *down below* or *down stairs*.

- The **penis** may be described as a *willy* (especially by children), *member, dick, prick, tool, John Thomas* (or occasionally *Johnny*) or other pet words including *todger*.

- The **prepuce** may be described as ***foreskin***, *helmet* or *hood*.

- **Testicles (testes)** may be referred to as *balls, bollocks* and *goolies*, and the **scrotum** as the *ball-bag* or just plain *bag*. A **hydrocoele** (*collection of fluid around a testis*) may be demonstrated by **transillumination** (*a torch test*).

Gynaecology

Anatomy

The **vagina** may be referred to as *up inside*, *down below*, *front bottom* or *passage*, *private* (*part*), *pussy*, *fanny*, *slit* or *birth canal*.

Clitoris may be abbreviated to *clit* and **labia** occasionally referred to as *flaps*.

The **cervix** is the *neck of the womb* and the **uterus** the *womb* or occasionally *box*.

Women aged 25–64 are invited to attend for the **NHS cervical screening programme** and understand that this involves passing a **speculum** (*small instrument*) and then having a **spatula** (*small and smooth wooden or plastic instrument*) inserted to *wipe* over the cervix to collect cells which are then examined under a microscope by a specialist. **Dyskaryosis** would be understood as *abnormal cells* and a **colposcopy** is a *closer examination* in the hospital **outpatients** (*clinic*).

Menstrual periods are referred to as *periods*, *time of the month*, *monthlies* or *being on* (my period).

Menorrhagia (*heavy periods*) may be caused by **fibroids** (*a muscular knot*) and **dysmenorrhea** (*painful periods*) is often abbreviated by patients to *dysmen*.

Intermenstrual bleeding is understood as *spotting* and **postcoital bleeding** as *bleeding after sex/intercourse*.

Such symptoms may merit further investigation including a **D&C** (*scrape*) or **hysteroscopy** (*further examination with a small instrument*), which may show, for example, **endometrial hyperplasia** (*overgrowth of the lining of the womb*).

Patients often attribute **gynaecological** (**gynae**) symptoms such as **PMT** to a *hormone imbalance*. The **menopause** is described as the *change* (*of life*) and the **vasomotor symptoms** would be described as *flushes* or *night sweats*, for which they may wish to take **hormone replacement therapy (HRT)**.

Breast screening

Women in the UK are taught about breast awareness and the NHS **mammography** (**breast screening**) programme invites women aged 50–64 to have an X-ray to detect breast cancer at an early stage.

Family planning/contraception

Communication

'What sort of contraception do you use?' is adequate for most occasions.

The **sheath** typically is referred to as a **condom** but may be referred to by brand such as **Durex**, the **diaphragm** is referred to as the **cap**, the intra-uterine contraceptive device (**IUCD**) as the **coil**, any **oral contraceptive** as **the pill** and a **vasectomy** is often the snip. Some other methods such as the **safe period** or **rhythm** method may be referred to as *taking precautions* and **coitus interruptus** as *we are very careful*, which amounts to *living dangerously*.

Pregnancy

Women who think that they might have *fallen* **pregnant** will report that they are *late* (with their period) and may have done a *home* **(pregnancy)** *test* which they may refer to by the proprietary brand such as *Clear Blue*. Women who are ***expecting*** (a baby) may describe *having a bun in the oven, being up the spout* or occasionally *up the junction*.

The **expected date of confinement/delivery (EDC/EDD)** (*due date*) is calculated from the first day of the **last menstrual period (LMP)** and may be confirmed by an **ultrasound scan** (*a painless test with a special camera using sound waves that shows a picture/* ***image*** *on a TV screen* (***monitor***)).

Women may suffer from morning sickness and other symptoms of pregnancy such as *feeling little 'un* (little one) *moving* and may describe the sensation of *blooming*, especially in the middle **trimester** (*third*) of pregnancy.

Occasionally problems during pregnancy are related to a problem with the **placenta** (*afterbirth*), for example **abruption** (*separation*). Following childbirth a number of new mothers experience **lability of mood** (*up and down*) and tearfulness (***baby blues***), which must be differentiated from postnatal depression.

The medical term **lactating** is understood as ***breast-feeding*** or ***nursing***.

Sexually transmitted infections (STIs)

Communication

When considering a STI, questions that might be asked by an IMG include:

- 'Do you have any discharge from the genitalia?'

But this could be abbreviated to **'Do you have any discharge?'** In the case of a man this would normally be taken as a **penile discharge** (from the urethra) and in the case of a woman it would be taken as a **vaginal discharge** rather than from the **urethra** (*front, water or outlet passage that drains urine from the bladder*).

Women may present complaining of having *thrush* **(candidiasis, monilia)**.

If men fear that they have **contracted** (*caught*) a sexually transmitted infection they may refer to it as a *dose* and specifically if it was **gonorrhoea** they may describe it as *the clap* and if **syphilis** *the pox*.

When enquiring about the risk of STIs some of the questions that an IMG might ask include:

- 'Do you believe in casual sex?'

- 'Do you have unprotected sex/intercourse?'

- 'What is your sexual preference?'

- 'How many partners have you had?' is likely to result in a defensive response.

But **'Do you practise safe sex?'** is probably more effective.

Patients with a suspected STI may self-refer to the **genito-urinary medicine (GUM) clinic**, which is often referred to as the ***special*** *clinic*, where they would be able to undertake diagnostic tests for conditions such as **HIV** as well as initiating **contact tracing**.

Sexual and relationship problems

Communication

Raising sexual matters with patients can be difficult and in both sexes many sexual problems may be associated with urinary symptoms.

- **'Are you in a stable (steady) relationship?'** or

- **'Do you/have you a (regular) partner?'**

It is considered to be more 'politically correct' to use the term **partner** than the terms boy/girl friend or husband or wife. However, it is reasonable, where appropriate, to ask whether patients are married and/or they have any children.

Patients are often reluctant to present with psycho-sexual problems but it is helpful to know some of the terms that they use to hide their embarrassment.

When a patient has **loss of libido** (*sex drive*) they may describe *going off* either *it* or *the other*, losing their *desire* or their *virility/manhood/masculinity* or having *no interest* (*in sex*), but if they are **having sex/intercourse** (*sleeping with someone, making love, getting laid, shagging*) they may have **anorgasmia** (*inability to climax/come*).

An **erection** may be described as having a *hard-on* and **erectile dysfunction** or ***impotence*** as *difficulty keeping it up, droop* (as in *brewer's droop* (due to the occupational hazards of drinking excess alcohol)).

Occasionally such sexual problems may be due to **a deficiency of androgens/testosterone** (*male sex hormone*).

Other sexual problems include **premature ejaculation** (*coming too soon*).

Some doctors might attempt a direct and closed question such as: **'How is your relationship with your partner?'**

When taking a sexual history questions that may be used by an IMG include:

- 'Are you sexing nicely?'

but **'How is your sex life?'** or **'Is your sex life enjoyable?'** are perfectly adequate for most occasions.

If a married person is having an extra-marital relationship it may be referred to as *having an affair* or *having a bit on the side* or alternatively *a fling* or *playing away from home*.

Same-sex relationships (*homosexuality*)

Gay is a term that is used to describe both male and female same-sex relationships but there are specific terms that are used for each gender, for example a woman may be referred to as being a *lesbian* or a *dyke* and a man as being a *homosexual, homo, ginger, puff/poof, queer,* or *shirt-lifter*. Some of these are derogatory terms that are more likely to be used by some heterosexuals. A **bisexual** person may have a partner of either gender.

In terms of homosexual sexual practice, drugs such as **amyl nitrite** (*poppers*) are occasionally used by some gay men to relax the anal sphincter and **anal intercourse** may be **penetrative** or **receptive**.

There are many terms used to describe a variety of sexual practices that may be volunteered when appropriate in the medical context, such as *rimming* (ano-oral contact) and *fisting*.

10 Muscular-skeletal system (*bones, joints and soft tissues*)

Children

Children may suffer from significant orthopaedic problems such as **congenital talipes equinovarus** (*club foot*) or **scoliosis** (*curvature of the spine*) and a number of other less serious problems including **in-toeing**, **bow legs**, **knock knees** or **flat feet**.

Hip problems include **developmental dysplasia of the hip (DDH)/congenital dislocation of the hip (CDH)** which is suspected clinically by the presence of a clunk rather than an audible click without **palpable** (*felt*) movement of the head of the femur.

When a child starts walking, DDH may present as a limp but in older children it is important to exclude **Perthé's disease** (**avascular necrosis** of the femoral head) explained as *damage to the top of the thigh bone caused by poor blood supply*; or a **slipped upper femoral epiphysis** (*slipped end part of long bone during growth*).

Trauma (*injuries*)

Patients who have suffered from serious trauma are managed by a **scoop and run** approach to getting the best available treatment in the shortest time possible.

Patients often self-refer to Accident and Emergency Departments with varying degrees of **trauma** (*injury*) including an **abrasion** (*graze*), a **laceration** (*cut*), a **haematoma** (*bruise*) or **fracture** (*broken or cracked bone* [the latter especially when it is a rib]). **Wounds** may **require** (*need*), firstly, **debridement** (*cleaning and tidying*) and secondly **suturing** (*stitching*) and finally **dressing**.

Patients often present with *strained muscles* or more specific problems such as a *sprained ankle* (**any ankle injury**), which they will explain as having *gone over on it* or less frequently *rolled it* (**an inversion injury**); or a (self-diagnosed) *frozen shoulder* (*inflammation in the joint causing stiffness*) although such patients often may have other problems such as **supraspinatus tendonitis** (*pain at the tip of the shoulder caused by inflammation in a leader/tendon*) resulting in a **painful arc**.

Following a **road traffic accident (RTA)** many patients will present with a *whiplash injury* (*strain of the ligaments holding the neck vertebrae together*), but some neck pain may be spontaneous in onset such as an **acute spasmodic torticollis (*wry neck*)**.

Aches and pains

Patients complain of having *a touch of lumbago* (*back ache*) or *rheumatism*, by which they mean *aching joints* (**arthralgia**). **Osteoarthrosis/osteoarthritis** is understood as *wear and tear* (**degeneration**) of the joints and **osteoporosis** as *brittle bone disease*.

Patients sometimes present complaining that they have '*put their back out*' and fear that they have ***slipped a disc*** (suffered a **prolapsed inter-vertebral disc**).

Soft tissue problems are common and, for example, patients may present with a variety of aches and pains that might relate to a **tendon** (*leader, guider*) problem, such as **lateral epicondylitis** (*tennis elbow*) or **medial epicondylitis** (*golfer's elbow*).

Polymyalgia rheumatica may be understood as *muscular rheumatism*.

Glossary of other useful muscular-skeletal terms:

- **Axilla:** *arm-pit*

- **Clavicle:** *collar-bone*

- **Femur:** *thigh-bone*

- **Olecranon bursitis:** *students' elbow*

- **Osteoporosis:** *brittle bone disease*

- **Patella:** *kneecap*

- **Plantar fasciitis:** *policeman's heel*

- **Prepatellar bursitis:** *house-maid's knee*

- **Sternum:** *breast-bone*

- **Vertebral column:** *spine*

- **Zygoma:** *cheek-bone*

Muscular-skeletal system (bones, joints and soft tissues)

11 Ophthalmological system (*eyes*)

An **ophthalmologist** is known as a *hospital eye specialist* but many patients will initially see a *high street optician* (who may also be an **optometrist**) for an ***eye check***, especially if they have a **refractive error** (*disorder in shape and size of the eye*).

The common refractive disorders are **hypermetropia** (long sight), **myopia** (short sight) and **astigmatism** (vertical or horizontal distortion of vision).

It is good practice to check the **visual acuity** (*eyesight*) in any patient with an eye problem and some patients enquire when they have *twenty-twenty vision* although they are disappointed to learn that the Snellen chart used in the UK assesses their vision using numbers such as 6/6.

Infants are assessed for **strabismus** (*squint/lazy eye*) but this is often difficult to exclude if there is a **broad epicanthus** (*wide bridge of nose and/or fold of skin at the inner angle of each eye*) and the diagnosis may require referral for an **orthoptic assessment** (*to assess the movements of the eyes*). The aims of treatment for squints in children are to correct any defect of visual acuity, achieve a satisfactory **cosmetic appearance** (*good appearance*) and ensure **binocular** (*using both eyes*) **vision**.

Patients may present complaining that they have *something in their eye* **(foreign body)** but sometimes they have a **corneal abrasion** (*scratch on the surface of the eye*), a **stye** (*infection in a lash hair follicle*), a **Meibomian cyst (chalazion)**, **blepharitis** (*inflammation of the lid*) or **conjunctivitis** (*red-eye*).

Occasionally patients will present with **epiphora** (*watering eye*) and, especially in the elderly, they may have an **ectropion** (*lid falling away from the eye*) or **entropion** (*lid turning inwards*).

Examination of the eyes may reveal **arcus senilis** (*white ring around the edge of the cornea*) or **xanthelasma** (*fatty deposits in the skin at the inner aspect of the eye*) and such patients may have a lipid disorder, although often it is found to be **physiological** (*normal*).

Some will be concerned by the appearances of *fatty deposits/blisters on the visible white of the eye* **(pinguecula)**, which really have no pathological consequence as opposed to the potentially more serious **pterygium** (*fold of tissue that may encroach on the cornea and affect vision*).

When patients complain of **episodic** (*intermittent*) **blurred vision** it is important to ask whether they also have **halos** (*rainbows around lights*) and *eye pain* to exclude **glaucoma** (*raised pressure in the eye*).

However, **floaters** are reported more frequently, especially against a pale background, and if there is no change in visual acuity they are not likely to be associated with serious eye disease, in contrast to a short-sighted person who suddenly has a change in visual acuity and who sees *sparks* or *stars*, who may have a **retinal detachment**.

Diplopia (*double vision*) may be associated with **systemic** (*generalised*) disease such as **thyroid disease** or **cerebro-vascular disease**.

Age-related problems include **presbyopia** (*long-sightedness*), **cataracts** (*clouding of the lenses*) or **macular degeneration**, for which some people are helped by low vision aids.

Visual impairment (*blindness* or *partial sight*) is **registered** by an **ophthalmologist** when the distance visual acuity is reduced to 3/60 or less or 6/60 or less, respectively, and confers a number of benefits such as access to **guide dogs** and to **talking books**.

12 Endocrine (*hormone*) system

The **pituitary gland** (*master gland*) produces a number of **hormones** (*chemical messengers*) that control other **glands** (*tissues that produce hormones*) so a pituitary deficiency (*failure to produce sufficient hormone*) will affect a number of target organs.

The **thyroid gland** may become enlarged producing a **goitre** and **myxoedema** (*an underactive thyroid gland*) may develop **insidiously** (*slowly and subtly*) causing the typical clinical picture, which may include **hypothermia** (*reduced body temperature*), while **thyrotoxicosis** (*an overactive thyroid gland*) may be associated with thyroid eye disease, including **lid retraction** (*white of the eye visible below the upper eyelid*) or **exophthalmos** (*prominent eyes caused by swelling of tissues behind the eyes*).

Communication

For example, in **diabetes mellitus**, the questions that an IMG might ask include:

- 'Are you having diabetes?'

- 'Are you fine for diabetes?'

But **'Do you suffer from diabetes?'** works better.

Diabetes mellitus is often referred to as *sugar diabetes* and patients may present with **polydipsia** (*increased thirst*) but often are concerned that they may be diabetic if they feel light-headed before meals, which is more likely to be due to **hypoglycaemia** (*low blood sugar/**glucose***).

A patient who suffers from type 1 diabetes mellitus may develop ***lipodystrophy*** (*thickening* or *pitting at the injection site*).

Occasionally metabolic problems are **iatrogenic** (*caused by doctors' treatment*) such as **hypernatraemia** (*too much salt in the blood*).

13 Dermatological system (*skin*)

Given that the skin is the biggest organ and that they can see it, patients often present with rashes (*spots*) which may be described as being ***red* (erythematous)**, ***itchy* (pruritic)**, ***hot*** and occasionally a self-diagnosis will be offered such as ***hives/nettle-rash* (papular urticaria)**, which is characterised by the presence of **papules** (*raised red spots*).

Congenital (*born with*) **lesions** or **birthmarks** include **a stork mark**, which is a flat, pinkish **capillary haemangioma** (*prominent small blood vessels in the skin*) at the nape of the neck, a **strawberry naevus** (*soft, raised, bright red prominent blood vessels in the skin*) and a **port-wine stain** (*flat purple patch caused by prominent small blood vessels which does not fade*).

Small **pigmented birthmarks (*moles*)** commonly develop after two years of age and a **Mongolian blue spot** is a large bluish-grey area most commonly over the **sacrum** (*lower back*) or buttocks.

Babies may be presented with rashes such as **milia** (*milk spots*), ***cradle cap* (seborrhoeic dermatitis)** or ***nappy rash* (ammoniacal dermatitis)**, which is usually confined to the skin in contact with a wet nappy – the **flexures** (*skin creases*) are spared as they don't come into contact with the urine.

Patients with young children are invariably worried about the possibility of **meningitis** (*inflammation of the lining of the brain*) when their children have any febrile illness associated with a rash and many will report that they have done the ***glass test***, which, if negative, means that it is a **blanching** and **non-purpuric** rash.

Dermatitis and/or **eczema** often result from sensitivity (*allergy*) to an **external** (*outside*) agent which leads to **inflammation** (*swelling*) of the skin which typically will cause ***irritation*** (*itch*) and if such a rash becomes infected then the wound may produce an **exudate**, in which case it would be described as *weeping*.

A condition such as **psoriasis** can be explained as comprising raised, red, scaling patches caused when the cells divide or multiply too quickly and the condition **relapses** and **remits** (*comes and goes*).

Skin infections are common and may include *cold sores* **(herpes simplex labialis)** or bacterial infections such as **impetigo** (*infectious skin condition*) or **cellulitis** (*a spreading tissue infection*).

Fungal infections include **tinea corporis** (*ringworm*), **tinea pedis** (*athlete's foot*) and **tinea cruris** (*jock itch*).

Pediculosis affecting the head hair in children (*nits and lice*) is **prevalent** (*common*) in children and in adults when affecting pubic hair may be referred to as *crabs or lice*.

***Teenagers* (adolescents)** frequently seek advice **(consult)** with concerns about their complexion and will describe the lesions of ***acne* (vulgaris)** graphically as *blackheads* **(comedones)**, *whiteheads* **(pustules)**, *zits* or *plukes*.

Patients often present with ***moles* (pigmented lesions)** and lumps, especially those which change, and are especially concerned about **malignant melanomas**, although **benign** (***non cancerous***) ***skin lumps* (tumours)** are much more common such as a **sebaceous (epidermoid) cyst** (*fluid-filled sac in a grease or natural oil producing gland*) or a **lipoma** (*fatty lump*).

Patients may present with **hirsuitism** (*increase in body hair*) or **alopecia** (*baldness, hair loss or thinning of hair*) and, less frequently, **hyperhidrosis** (*excessive sweating*).

Occasionally patients will present with a rash that they may relate to their *nerves* **(neurodermatitis)** and others may have a **photosensitivity** (*increased sensitivity to sunlight*).

14 Physical examination

Doctors are required to assess the condition of a patient by conducting an appropriate examination to confirm or disprove their working diagnosis and to address the patient's concern.

Communication

For example, in the **examination of the breast** (*boob*) in a patient who has discovered a lump, although the principles apply for any physical examination, a commentary is often given by an IMG to an observing examiner such as:

- 'I'd like to ensure privacy.'

However, it is more important to address and explain the nature of the examination to the patient.
    Statements that have been used by IMGs include:

- 'I will be feeling for your breasts.'

- 'I'd like to examine your torso.'

- 'We need to feel (palpate) your breasts.'

- 'I'd like to examine/palpate/feel your breasts.'

But **'Is it alright if (May) I examine your breasts?'** would generally be preferable. An IMG would normally ask: **'Would you like a chaperone?'**, which is perfectly appropriate.
    When subsequently directing patients, questions that an IMG might ask include:

- 'Please will you undress above your waist.'

- 'Please take off your clothes from the waist above.'

- 'Could you undress from the waist above?'

But **'Would you mind removing your top?'** works just as well.

An IMG might proceed to ask questions including:

- 'Which side (or where) do you get this feeling of a lump?'

But **'Which side is the lump on?'** is more succinct and **'Please can you show me where the lump is?'** is probably the best approach.
    It is helpful to explain to the patient the nature of the examination and to warn them about any potential discomfort. Examples of the reassurance given by an IMG include:

- 'I will hurt you as little as possible.'

- 'This may feel a bit ticklish.'

But **'This may cause some discomfort'**, followed where appropriate by **'Please let me know at any time if you wish me to stop'** would work just as well.

A commentary for the benefit of the examiner is often required for the purposes of an examination and this may include, on inspection:

- **'The breasts are pendulous.'**

- **'There is asymmetry of the breasts.'**

- **'The breasts are asymmetric or asymmetrical'** (if they are).

- **'There are no visible veins/scars/excoriations'** (signs of excoriation).

- **'The nipples are not inverted** (*turned in*) **or retracted'.**

- **'There is no puckering or tethering.'**

- **'I shall examine the breast in a clockwise manner.'**

'There are no swellings' is better expressed as: **'There are no palpable masses/lumps.'**

If a breast lump is present, a description should be given such as: **'The *swelling* (mass/ lump) measures 3 cm in diameter and has a smooth surface. It is not attached to the chest wall and is mobile. There is no nipple discharge.'**

Examination of the **axillae** (*armpits or under-arms*) may reveal anterior apical lymph glands (nodes).

However, while this approach is appropriate for the purposes of presenting the clinical findings to an examiner, in normal clinical practice it would be more appropriate to explain the findings and management plan to the patient, incorporating their preferences where appropriate.

At the end of a patient's physical examination an IMG may end with statements such as:

- 'You've been very co-operative.'

- 'Was it too bad for you?'

- 'That's very nice.'

- 'That's (very) fine.' or

- 'Thank you.'

But this is not appropriate and it may be better to 'safety net' and ensure that the patient returns as appropriate or to ask them if there is anything else that they need to discuss for example by asking questions such as:

- **'Do you have any other concerns?'**

- **'Is there anything else that you would like to discuss?'**

- **'Do you have any further questions which you feel that I have not answered?'**

- **'Is there anything else important that we have not discussed?'**

15 Management

Drug treatment

Having established a **definitive** (*accurate/correct*) diagnosis and made a **management plan**, the doctor would be expected to use appropriate prescribing behaviour, which may include **giving advice** or **issuing a prescription**.

Care should be taken to use simple language when describing **medications** (*drugs or medicines*) that are **prescribed** (*ordered, written-up*) by a doctor, **dispensed** (*issued*) by a **pharmacist (*chemist*)** or bought **over the counter (OTC)**, including, for example, in terms of routes of administration.

Examples include: **topically** may need to be explained as *apply to the skin*, **sublingually** as *under the tongue*, **lozenges/pastilles** as *sucked like throat sweets*, **orally** as *swallowed by mouth*, **inhaled** as *breathed in*, **nebulised** as *turned into a mist*, **injected** (*a needle*) by the following routes: **intramuscular** (*into a muscle*), **subcutaneous** (*under the skin*) or **intravenous** (*into a vein*). An **intravenous infusion** is understood as a ***drip***.

The word ***liquid*** is understood for **suspension**, **syrup**, or **linctus**.

The 'pill' is reserved specifically for the **contraceptive pill**.

Patients attend for **routine immunisations** or **travel vaccinations** which may be generically referred to as *jabs*, *shots*, *needles* or *boosters* (when appropriate).

Patients occasionally volunteer that they may be ***allergic*** to some drugs, especially antibiotics, but the term allergy is used somewhat loosely to include minor ***adverse/side effects*** such as diarrhoea. Clearly it is important to clarify whether there is a history of **anaphylaxis** (*serious or severe allergic reaction*).

The purpose of a medication may need to be explained, for example, a **prophylactic** could be described as a *preventer* or *protector*, such using an **inhaler** (*puffer, spray, pump*) for steroids in asthma (*brown inhaler*); and a **symptomatic treatment** as a *reliever* or *rescue treatment*, such as a **bronchodilator** (*drug to open up airways, blue inhaler*).

For specific conditions such as treatment of **malignancy (*cancer*)** it is helpful to be able to reassure a patient that they will be given adequate **analgesia** (*pain relief*) with **analgesics** (*pain killers*). Where appropriate they may have **chemotherapy** with **cytotoxic drugs** (*drugs which kill rapidly dividing cancer cells*) which may have **adverse** (*side*) effects such as **agranulocytosis or neutropenia** (*decrease in white blood cells*) that may result in them being **immunocompromised** (*having weakened resistance to infections*). However, some **tumours (*cancers*)** may be **resistant** (*difficult to treat*) to such drugs and may require **radiotherapy** (*X-ray treatment*).

Other helpful terms which are used in prescribing:

- **Concentration:** *strength*.
- **Discontinue:** *stop*.
- **Expiry (date):** *use by*.

Surgery

Minor surgery may include a number of procedures such as **cryotherapy** (*freezing*) using **liquid nitrogen (LN2)** to remove lesions such as *warts*.

Other minor procedures such as **aspiration** (*withdrawing fluid, sucking out*), **incision and drainage (I&D)** (*lancing*) of an **abscess**, *carbuncle* (*boil*) or **curettage** (*scraping*) and **diathermy** (*heat sealing* by an electrical instrument) by **excision** (*cutting out*) of *lumps and bumps*, and typically these would be done under a **local anaesthetic** (*freezing the skin*).

Major surgery (*operations*) would generally require a **general anaesthetic** (*pain-free sleep*) and might initially involve a **laparotomy** (*exploratory*) before proceeding with a definitive procedure such as an **excision** (*cutting out*) or repair of a **lesion**.

The general principles of surgical procedures are similar across surgical specialities but examples are given for urological surgery.

Patients may present with, for example, **acute retention of urine** (*inability to pass urine/wee*) and would be treated by insertion of a self-retaining **urethral catheter** (*tube passed into bladder to drain urine*).

Investigation typically would involve a **cystoscopy** using a traditional **cystoscope**, which is an instrument to look in the urethra and bladder and is essentially a *long* (*and rigid*) *telescope incorporating a light*, or a **flexible cystoscope** using **fibreoptics** (*a telescope with a powerful light shining down glass fibres*).

A urethral stricture may be treated by inserting **sounds** or **bougies** (*dilators*) and if this fails a **urethrotomy** (*slit or cut in the narrowing of the urethra*) may be performed. However, this may give only short-lived relief and it may be necessary to proceed to some form of **urethroplasty** (*a plastic procedure in which a full thickness of skin is inlaid to keep it permanently open*).

A **biopsy** (*sample of tissue removed for further examination*) would be taken from any **lesion** (*abnormality including due to disease or injury*).

Operations that might be done on the kidney include a **nephrectomy** (*removal of a kidney*); a **pyeloplasty** to relieve **pelviureteric junction (PUJ) obstruction** (*plastic operation to relieve a blockage at the outlet from the kidney*); a **nephrostomy** (*a cut to provide a temporary measure to relieve a temporary blockage to the ureter*); a **transplantation** of a donor kidney.

A simple **cystotomy** (*cutting the bladder open*) would be performed to remove a stone that was too large to remove by **litholapaxy** (*through a cystoscope*).

A **partial cystectomy** may be done for rare and isolated bladder tumours on the **vault** (*arched roof/top*). Following a **total cystectomy** (*removal of the bladder* for cancer) a urinary diversion is required using for example an **ileal conduit** in which the *ureters are implanted into an isolated loop of small bowel* which would depend on having an ileal **stoma** (*bag on the abdominal wall*).

The **prostate** may be removed either by a **transurethral resection (TURP)** (*internally*) using a **resectoscope** or by an open operation (*through a cut in the abdomen*).

Laparoscopic procedures are often understood as *keyhole surgery*.

16 Death and related issues

Risk

Doctors are often asked to communicate **prognosis** (*outlook*) or risks of treatment or non-treatment to patients and they may use terms such as **number needed to treat** (*number of patients who need to be treated to prevent a single additional adverse outcome*) or **5-year survival rates**.

It is helpful to be able to explain such concepts in terms that the patient may understand, for example, **a mortality rate** could be explained as *the chance of dying from a particular condition*. It's often difficult for a patient to work out their individual risk from statistical odds and some doctors will resort to illustrative terms that attempt to put a risk in perspective such as being **as rare as hens' teeth** (which don't exist) would mean that the chance is so small that they could (virtually) ignore it.

Death

Some patients may sign a **living will** or **advance directive** to state their wishes about medical treatment should they develop a serious illness.

Death still remains a taboo subject for many patients and their relatives and a number of euphemisms are in common use to describe the deceased, especially *passed away* but also *passed on, expired, gone to sleep* or more irreverently having *kicked the bucket* or *popped their clogs*.

Following the death of a patient a death certificate may be issued unless there is some reason why the case should be referred to the **coroner** (or **Procurator Fiscal** in Scotland). Funeral directors make the funeral arrangements and the majority of the deceased are cremated (requiring two doctors to sign a cremation certificate) rather than having a burial.

17 And finally . . .

Pitfalls

Some of the pitfalls for doctors in using unfamiliar idiom lie in using it in the wrong context or when it isn't quite delivered accurately, for example: 'Have you had "flies" in your stomach?' when 'butterflies' were intended or 'When you have passed the "honey" period' when 'honeymoon' was intended.

The term **diabetic nurse**, for example, could be taken to mean a nurse who suffers from diabetes mellitus, although the term would more usually be used to describe a nurse who specialises in the care of patients suffering from diabetes mellitus. Such confusion can be avoided by adopting the precise term **diabetic specialist nurse**.

Similarly, 'seen by a cooperative doctor' may be interpreted as a patient attending a particularly compliant doctor or that a patient was seen by a doctor at an out-of-hours co-operative on-call centre.

Pronunciation *(see also* Module 30: Confusing words . . . and Module 32: Phrasal verbs)

The English language has a number of words that are difficult to pronounce and those that are especially troublesome for some IMGs include:

- migraine: may be pronounced m-ee-graine or m-eye-graine

- debris: is pronounced with a silent 's' that is as 'debri'

- lipids: is pronounced lipids, the first 'i' as in 'bit' and not l-eye-pids

- tethering: a difficult word to pronounce correctly as it is often expressed as tithering or teethering but tethering is pronounced with the first 'e' as in the word 'best'

- vomit: V can be a difficult letter to pronounce but it is worth trying to master the V as in 'vowel', to avoid pronouncing 'vomit' as 'womit'.

18 Medicine in the UK

Structure of NHS services

The **National Health Service** (NHS) provides comprehensive healthcare free at the point of delivery, funded by the state through direct taxation. The **Secretary of State for Health** is the head of the **Department of Health** (DoH) and advises the government on healthcare policy.

Primary care services

Traditionally, care is accessible in primary care from a **general practitioner (GP)**, who typically works in a **group practice** with a **primary healthcare team** and has a registered list of patients for whom he will provide a range of services. In addition, **NHS Direct** offers nurse-led telephone advice to patients.

Currently vocational training for general practice involves two years of recognised hospital SHO posts and one year as a **General Practice Registrar (GPR)** attached to a recognised training practice, following which a certificate of prescribed experience is issued and a GP may apply for a post as a GP principal or non-principal, which would be attached to one or more practices on a sessional or a salaried basis.

Secondary care is typically provided by a **district general hospital** (DGH) and direct access is available only through accident and emergency (A&E) or emergency departments, to which patients may self-refer. However, in the majority of cases a GP will refer a patient for secondary care, although in the case of an emergency a patient or their relative may dial 999 and be taken to hospital by a state-funded ambulance.

Other community care includes nursing, child, maternity, terminal and mental health services, which may be provided by community-based specialists, specialist nurses and GPs.

Social services are responsible for the support of potentially vulnerable groups, such as the elderly, homeless or victims of abuse, and the social security system pays (financial) benefits to the needy.

Working in a DGH

A DGH typically will offer a full range of acute services for a specified population of patients and is managed by a trust which comprises a board headed by a chief executive with managers and clinical directors providing a clinical management interface.

At present hospital medical staff comprises career grades, including consultants, associate specialists and staff grades, and training grades – namely specialist registrars, (spR), senior house officers (SHO) and pre-registration house officers (PRHO).

Currently a review of the structure of the training grades is taking place but at present the **PRHO** has only provisional registration and clinical responsibility under supervision for one year; an **SHO** would be undertaking basic specialist training for 2–3 years, following which they may apply for a **spR** post undertaking higher specialist training, lasting from 4–6 years depending on the speciality. Once they have gained their **Certificate of Completion of Specialist Training (CCST)** they are entitled to apply for the position of a consultant.

A **staff grade** provides an essential role in the hospital medical team but the post is not recognised as a training post, which makes it difficult to obtain the CCST, although it is possible to progress to become an **associate specialist**.

Management of non-acute and primary care services

A similar management structure exists for both non-acute services such as mental health and for a **Primary Care Organisation (PCO)**, which has a **services management team (SMT)**. In addition, a PCO has a **Professional Executive Committee (PEC)**, which includes representation from nurses, dentists, opticians, pharmacists as well as GPs who advise on local health issues.

The structure of healthcare organisations is broadly similar throughout the UK but there are some regional differences between England, Scotland, Wales and Northern Ireland.

Under the new Contract, the PCO is responsible for providing out of hours (OOH) cover.

Other important organisations

The General Medical Council (GMC) is the regulatory body that is responsible for issues such as registration, revalidation, professional conduct, performance and administration of the PLAB exam. The function of the GMC can be summarised as 'protecting patients and guiding doctors' and this is described in a number of documents such as *Duties of a Doctor* and *Good Medical Practice*.

The **British Medical Association** (BMA) is the doctors' professional organisation and produces the weekly **British Medical Journal (BMJ)**, in which most job vacancies are advertised.

The **Medical Defence Union (MDU)** is the largest of a few organisations that provide professional indemnity as an insurance against cases of medical malpractice.

The **Postgraduate Medical Education Training Board (PMETB)** is a new body that advises on the principles and the standards of postgraduate medical assessment and will take over the function of the **Specialist Training Authority (STA)** and the **Joint Committee for Postgraduate Training for General Practice (JCPTGP)**.

The **Deaneries** are responsible for implementing and ensuring the standards of training of doctors.

Part Two

1 Condition

A Look at these sentences. They all use 'if'. Rewrite each sentence, replacing 'if' with the words in **bold**. You may need to remove some of the other words.

1 You can borrow my dictionary if you return it before you go home.
providing that

2 You can't go to university if you don't have good grades.
unless

3 Pollution will get worse if we continue to live in a throwaway society.
as long as

4 Many developed countries are willing to waive the Third World debt if the money is reinvested in education and medicine
on condition that

5 Some countries will never be able to rectify their deficits even if they work very hard.
no matter how

6 Computers are difficult things to understand, even if you read a lot of books about them.
however many

7 Crime is a problem, even if you go to relatively safe countries.
wherever

B Now rewrite each sentence beginning with the words in **bold**. For example:

Providing that you return it before you go home, you can borrow my dictionary.

C Complete these sentences using an appropriate word or expression from above and your own ideas.

1 British universities will accept students from abroad . . .
2 Working for a large company can be a fulfilling experience . . .
3 Most banks are happy to lend customers money . . .
4 The government will reduce income tax . . .
5 The environmental situation will continue to worsen . . .
6 There will always be long waiting lists at our hospitals . . .
7 Travelling helps you understand more about the world around you . . .

D Some nouns can be used to express condition. Complete these sentences 1–3 with one of the words from A, B or C.

1 Being able to drive is one of the . . . . of the job of salesman.
   A. prerequirements   **B. prerequisites**   **C. prescriptions**

2 Before you accept a job, it is important that you agree with the . . . . of the contract.
   A. conditionals   **B. conditions**   **C. conditioners**

3 It is a . . . . of the university that you attend an interview.
   A. requirement   **B. requisite**   **C. requiem**

Look at the pairs of sentences in 1–20 and choose a verb from the box which can be used with both sentences. In some cases, the meaning of the verb may change slightly. Then use a dictionary to find other objects which can be used with the verbs.

| • adapt • adjust • alter • cure • demote • disappear • dissolve |
| • exchange • expand • fade • increase • promote • reduce |
| • renew • renovate • replace • swell • switch • transform • vary |

1	We need to . . . . these cars so disabled people can drive them.	The country found it hard to . . . . to the new government
2	If the trousers are too tight, take them back to the shop and ask them to . . . . them.	He found it hard to . . . . to living in a tropical country.
3	You must . . . . the voltage or the system will blow up.	He decided to . . . . his appearance by having plastic surgery.
4	Our bills will be less if we . . . . from gas to electricity.	They had to . . . . flights at Heathrow Airport
5	You can't . . . . the terms of the contract once it has been signed.	He wants to . . . . his appearance.
6	It will help your digestion if you . . . . your diet.	Prices of flats . . . . from a few thousand to millions of pounds.
7	We need to . . . . our pounds for dollars.	You can usually . . . . goods which are faulty if you show the receipt.
8	We have had to . . . . our sales force to cope with the extra demand.	Water will . . . . when it is frozen.
9	The price of oil will . . . . next year.	Most bosses refuse to . . . . salaries when they are asked.
10	The management decided to . . . . the company and sell the offices.	. . . . the sugar in boiling water

11	More and more people are moving to cities to . . . . the populations there	The wasp sting caused his leg to . . . . up.
12	The market for typewriters will probably . . . . completely in the next few years.	The police are baffled by the increasing number of people who . . . . each year.
13	The old contract ran out and we had to . . . . it.	Many people argue that it's futile to . . . . old hostilities.
14	They have received funds to . . . . the old buildings.	We need to . . . . the central heating as it is old and worn out.
15	The boss offered to . . . . him from salesman to manager.	Our main aim is to . . . . tourism in the country.
16	They wanted to . . . . me from manager to salesperson.	If we . . . . you, you will lose a large part of your salary.
17	If you wash it too much, the colour will	We watched the islands . . . . away into the distance.
18	The company decided to . . . . the permanent staff with freelancers.	You must . . . . the books on the shelf when you have finished with them.
19	The doctors were unable to . . . . her illness.	. . . . the meat in salt water for between three and five days.
20	Governments are trying to . . . . pollution.	The best way to save money is to . . . . the number of staff.

A Look at the four tables below. These show demographic trends in four different countries between 1996 and 2000. The numbers on the left and right of each table show the number of people in millions. Using the information in these tables, match sentences 1–13 with the appropriate country. Use the words and expressions in **bold** to help you.

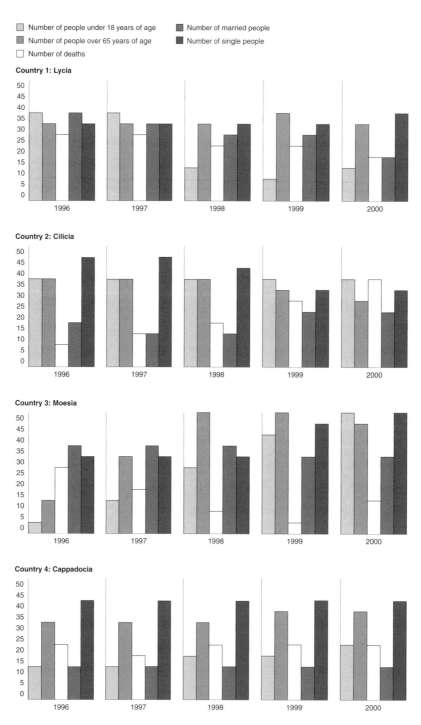

1 In which two countries was there a **considerable discrepancy** between married and single people between 1996 and 1998?

2 In which country was there a **constant** and **considerable discrepancy** between married and single people over the five-year period?

3 In which country was there a **sudden** and **noticeable difference** between those under 18 and those over 65 in 1998?

4 In which country did the number of under-18s **rise dramatically** between 1996 and 2000?

5 In which country did the number of under-18s **increase slightly** between 1996 and 2000?

6 In which country did the number of over-65s **go up sharply** between 1996 and 1998?

7 In which country did the number of married people **decline** over the five-year period?

8 In which country did the number of deaths **decrease significantly** between 1996 and 1999?

9 In which country was there a **slight decline** in the number of married people between 1998 and 1999?

10 In which country was there a **sharp drop** in the number of under-18s between 1997 and 1998?

11 In which country was there a **slight reduction** in the number of deaths over the five-year period?

12 In which country was there a **significant increase** in the number of deaths between 1998 and 2000?

13 In which country did the number of deaths **remain constant** over the five-year period?

B Now look at the table below, which shows the changes in economic activity in a town over a period of five years. The figures on the left and right show the number of people involved in these activities, in thousands. Write your own sentences to describe the situation in the town regarding the number of:

1 people employed in industry between 1996 and 2000.

2 people employed in retail between 1996 and 2000.

3 people employed in public services between 1999 and 2000.

4 people employed in tourism between 1996 and 2000.

5 unemployed between 1998 and 2000.

6 people employed in industry compared with those in tourism in 1996.

7 people employed in industry between 1998 and 1999.

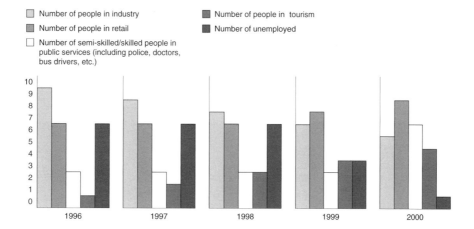

4 How something works

A Look at these sentences and decide which object is being described in each one. Use the words in **bold** to help you. You will find the objects hidden in the word grid at the bottom of the page.

1 The most important part of this object is a strip of two different metals, one on top of the other. As they **heat up**, both metals **expand**, but one does it faster than the other. The strip **bends** and **connects** with a switch, which **turns off** the power supply. When the strip **cools down**, the metals **contract** and the switch is **disconnected**. (1 word)

2 This object has several **component parts**, most of which are made of plastic. A disc inserted into the object **spins** quickly. At the same time a thin beam of light **strikes** the disc and **converts** digital symbols into sounds. These sounds can be **increased** or **decreased** in volume by means of a button or dial. (3 words)

3 Liquid and gas are **compressed** in a hard metal tube. This can be **released** by **pushing** or **squeezing** a button which **opens** a valve. When the liquid-gas combination **leaves** the tube and is mixed with oxygen, it rapidly **expands**. (1 word)

4 This object is mainly **made of** aluminium. As it **moves** forward, air **flows** over two horizontal sections. As it **accelerates**, a vacuum is **formed** over the horizontal sections and the object is pulled into the air by the force of this vacuum. (1 word)

5 This object consists of two main parts; one is made mainly of plastic and metal, the other is made mainly of glass. Light **enters** the glass section and a small door in the device **opens** up when a button is **pressed**. At the same time, a smaller window called an *aperture* **adjusts** itself to control the amount of light. The light is then **absorbed** by a sheet of plastic coated in a special chemical. An image is **formed** and this can then be **processed** and **developed** into a two-dimensional paper-based object. (1 word)

6 A sharp blade inside a plastic container **rotates** very quickly. It **chops** or **grinds** anything it touches, which we can then use to **produce** soup, sauces and dressing. (2 words)

7 This is a very simple object which originated in China. A small piece of paper is **lit** with a match. It **burns** away until the flame **ignites** the chemical compound inside a cardboard tube. The result is a display of light and colour. (1 word)

Q	C	A	R	E	N	G	I	N	E	W	E	R	T	T	Y	U
A	S	D	F	G	H	J	K	L	Z	X	C	V	B	O	N	M
B	A	L	L	P	O	I	N	T	P	E	N	A	Q	A	C	W
Q	W	E	R	F	O	O	D	P	R	O	C	E	S	S	O	R
B	T	Y	U	I	O	P	A	D	S	A	G	R	K	T	M	J
I	A	M	N	B	K	E	T	T	L	E	V	O	C	E	P	T
C	E	C	X	Z	L	K	J	H	G	F	D	S	S	R	U	H
Y	R	S	A	P	O	I	U	Y	T	R	E	O	E	W	T	E
C	O	M	P	A	C	T	D	I	S	C	P	L	A	Y	E	R
L	P	L	K	J	H	G	F	D	S	A	Q	W	E	R	R	M
E	L	I	G	H	T	B	U	L	B	M	N	B	V	C	X	O
C	A	M	E	R	A	I	F	I	R	E	W	O	R	K	U	S
L	N	K	J	H	G	F	D	S	A	Q	W	E	R	T	Y	T
T	E	L	E	V	I	S	I	O	N	T	Y	U	I	O	P	A
M	I	C	R	O	W	A	V	E	O	V	E	N	N	G	E	T

B There are nine more objects hidden in the grid. Choose four of them and write a brief description of how they work, using the bold words and expressions above.

5 Writing a letter

A Below, you will see eleven common situations that people encounter when they are writing a formal letter. Choose the sentence or phrase (A, B or C) that would be most appropriate in each situation.

1 You are writing a letter to the headteacher of a school or college, but you don't know their name. How do you begin your letter?
   A. Dear headteacher   **B. Dear Sir/Madam**   **C. Dear Sir**

2 You have received a letter from the manager of a company which buys computer components from your company, and you are now replying. What do you say?
   A. Thank you for your letter.
   B. Thanks a lot for your letter.
   C. It was great to hear from you.

3 You recently stayed in a hotel and were very unhappy with the service you received. You are now writing to the manager. What do you say?
   A. I had a horrible time at your hotel recently.
   B. I would like to say that I am unhappy about your hotel.
   C. I would like to complain about the service I received at your hotel recently.

4 You have sent a letter of application to a college, together with your curriculum vitae, which the college requested. What do you say in the letter to explain that your curriculum vitae is attached?
   A. You asked for my curriculum vitae, so here it is.
   B. As you can see, I've enclosed my curriculum vitae.
   C. As you requested, I enclose my curriculum vitae.

5 You have applied for a job, but you would like the company to send you more information. What do you say?
   A. I would be grateful if you would send me more information.
   B. I want you to send me more information.
   C. Send me some more information, if you don't mind.

6 In a letter you have written to a company, you tell them that you expect them to reply. What do you say?
   A. Write back to me soon, please.
   B. Please drop me a line soon.
   C. I look forward to hearing from you soon.

7 In a letter you have written, you want the recipient to do something and are thanking them in advance of their action. What do you say?
   A. Thank you for your attention in this matter.
   B. Thanks for doing something about it.
   C. I am gratified that you will take appropriate action.

8 The company you work for has received an order from another company and you are writing to them to acknowledge the order and let them know when you can deliver. What do you say?
   A. About the order you sent on 12 January for . . .
   B. I would like to remind you of the order you sent on 12 January for . . .
   C. I refer to your order of 12 January.

9 In a letter, you explain that the recipient can contact you if they want more information. What do you say?
   A. Give me a call if you want some more information.
   B. If you would like any more information, please do not hesitate to contact me.
   C. If you would like any more information, why not get in touch?

10 You began a letter with the recipient's name (e.g., Dear Mr. Perrin). How do you end the letter?
   A. Yours faithfully   **B. Yours sincerely**   **C. Best wishes**

11 You did not begin the letter with the recipient's name (see number 1 above). How do you end the letter?
   A. Yours faithfully   **B. Yours sincerely**   **C. Best wishes**

B Look at these sentences and decide if they are true or false.

1 Formal letters are always longer than informal letters.

2 In a formal letter it is acceptable to use colloquial English, slang and idioms.

3 In a formal letter it is acceptable to use contractions (e.g. I've instead of I have)

4 In a formal letter you should include your name and address at the top of the page.

5 In a formal letter, you should always write the date in full (e.g., 1 April 2000 and not 1/4/00).

6 In a formal letter, you should always put your full name (e.g., James Harcourt and not J. Harcourt) after your signature at the bottom of the letter.

7 Formal letters do not need to be broken into paragraphs. It is acceptable to write them as one continuous paragraph.

6 Presenting an argument

A Read the text below, in which somebody is trying to decide whether to go straight to university from school, or spend a year travelling around the world. Put their argument into the correct order, using the key words and expressions in **bold** to help you. The first one and last one have been done for you.

A I'm really in two minds about what to do when I leave school. Should I go straight to university or should I spend a year travelling around the world? (1)

B **It is often said that** knowledge is the key to power, and I cannot disagree with this.

C **On the one hand**, I would experience lots of different cultures.

D Unfortunately, **another point is that** if I spent a year travelling I would need a lot of money.

E And I'm not alone in this opinion. **Many consider** a sound career and a good salary to be an important goal.

F **However**, it could be argued that I would also meet lots of interesting people while I was travelling.

G **Secondly**, if I go straight to university, I'll learn so many things that will help me in my future life.

H **First of all**, there are so many benefits to going straight to university.

I But **I believe that** it would be easy to make a bit while I was travelling, giving English lessons or working in hotels and shops.

J **Moreover**, I'll be able to take part in the social activities that the university offers, and meet lots of new friends who share the same interests.

K **The most important point is that** the sooner I get my qualifications, the quicker I'll get a job and start earning.

L **Nevertheless**, these inconveniences would be an inevitable part of travelling and would be greatly outweighed by the other advantages.

M **In my opinion**, starting work and making money is one of the most important things in life.

N **On the other hand**, I could end up suffering from culture shock, homesickness and some strange tropical diseases.

O **Furthermore**, if I spent a year travelling, I would learn more about the world.

P All right, I've made my mind up. Now, where's my nearest travel agency? (16)

B Using the key words and expressions in **bold** from the last exercise, present an argument for *one* of the following issues:

1 A government's main priority is to provide education for its people.

2 The only way to save the environment is for governments to impose strict quotas on the energy we use (for example, by restricting car ownership, limiting the water we use).

3 Satisfaction in your job is more important than the money you earn.

4 Living in a town or city is better than living in the countryside.

5 It is our responsibility to help or look after those less fortunate than ourselves (for example, the homeless, the mentally ill).

7 Location

A Look at this diagram and complete the sentences below using the expressions in the box. In some cases, more than one answer is possible.

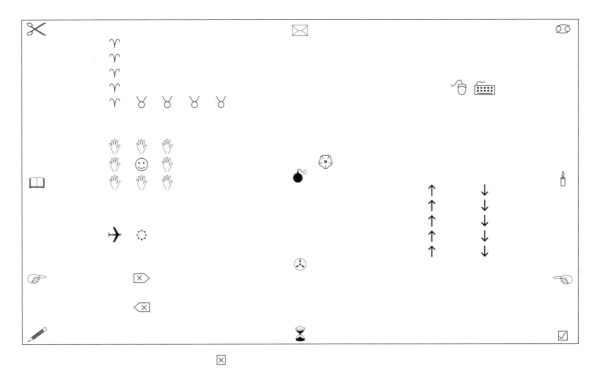

- ... directly opposite ...
- ... in close proximity to ...
- ... at the bottom of ...
- ... surrounded by ...
- ... exactly in the middle of ...
- ... halfway between ...
- ... at right angles to/perpendicular to ...
- ... on the left-hand side of ...
- ... in the top right-hand corner of ...
- ... on the right-hand side of ...
- ... to the left of ...
- ... in the bottom right-hand corner of ...
- ... in the top left-hand corner of ...
- ... stands outside ...
- ... in the bottom left-hand corner of ...
- ... roughly in the middle of ...
- ... parallel to ...
- ... at the top of ...
- ... to the right of ...

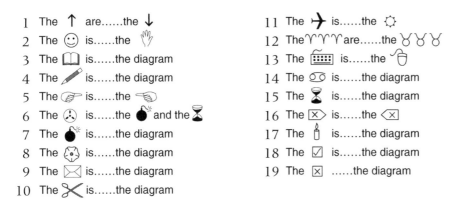

60

Location

B   How well do you know your country? Write the name of a city, town, village or island which . . .

1   . . . is situated in the middle of your country.
2   . . . is built on the slopes of a mountain.
3   . . . is located on the coast.
4   . . . stands on a cape or peninsula.
5   . . . is built on the edge of a river or lake.
6   . . . is a two-hour journey by car or bus from the capital.
7   . . . is a short distance off the coast.
8   . . . is about 10 miles (approximately 16 kilometres) from your home town.

Don't forget to keep a record of the words and expressions that you have learnt, review your notes from time to time and try to use new vocabulary items whenever possible.

8 Contrast and comparison

Complete these sentences with the most appropriate word or expression from A, B or C.

1 The two machines . . . . considerably. One has an electric motor, the other runs on oil.
   A. differ   **B. differentiate**   **C. differential**

2 The . . . . in weather between the north and the south of the country is very noticeable.
   A. comparison   **B. contrast**   **C. compare**

3 Many people cannot . . . . between lemon juice and lime juice.
   A. differ   **B. differentiate**   **C. contrast**

4 Children must be taught to . . . . between right and wrong.
   A. differ   **B. contrast**   **C. distinguish**

5 There is a . . . . between being interested in politics and joining a political party.
   A. distinguish   **B. distinctive**   **C. distinction**

6 Can you tell the . . . . between a good boss and a bad one?
   A. difference   **B. differentiate**   **C. contrast**

7 The management must not . . . . between male and female applicants.
   A. differ   **B. contrast**   **C. discriminate**

8 Asia covers a huge area. . . . . , Europe is very small.
   A. By way of contrast **B. By ways of comparing**   **C. By similar means**

9 The new model of car is very . . . . to the old one.
   A. same   **B. similar**   **C. common**

10 Her political opinions are . . . . to mine.
   A. same   **B. exactly**   **C. identical**

11 Some political parties have such similar manifestos that they are difficult to . . . .
   A. tell apart   **B. say apart**   **C. speak apart**

12 My friends and I enjoy doing many of the same things. In that respect, we have a lot . . . .
   A. in similar   **B. in particular**   **C. in common**

13 There seems to be a large . . . . between the number of people employed in service industries, and those employed in the primary sector.
   A. discriminate   **B. discretion**   **C. discrepancy**

14 British and Australian people share the same language, but in other respects they are as different as . . . .
   A. cats and dogs   **B. chalk and cheese**   **C. salt and pepper**

15 Britain's economy is largely based on its industry, ... a few hundred years ago it was an agrarian country.
   A. wherefore   **B. whereas**   **C. whereby**

9 Joining/becoming part of something bigger

The sentences below all contain a word or expression in **bold** which is related to joining two or more things, sometimes with the result of becoming part of something bigger. However, the words and expressions have all been put into the wrong sentence. Put them into their correct sentence. In some cases, more than one answer is possible.

A Move the verbs into the right sentences.

1 His salary is **merged** to the cost of living, and increases on an annual basis.
2 The International Book Association **blended** with Universal Press in 1999 to form the International Press.
3 To get a better finish, he **swallowed up** the two paints together.
4 The firm **integrated** with its main competitor in the battle to win more customers.
5 The suggestions from all the committees were **took over** into the main proposal.
6 The immigrants faced hostility when they were first **incorporated** into the community.
7 A lot of students had problems before they **amalgamated** into college life.
8 When the large international college **got together** the smaller school, a lot of people lost their jobs.
9 The students **linked** one evening and decided to protest about their situation.
10 A large international company **assimilated** our firm last month and started making immediate changes.

B Move the nouns into the right sentences.

1 The **alloy** between England and France came close to breaking down many times during the nineteenth century.
2 The **synthesis** between England and Scotland is over 300 years old.
3 The company has ten directors who provide a **blend** of different expertise.
4 Brass is a well-known **alliance** of copper and zinc.
5 Water is a **coalition** of hydrogen and oxygen.
6 The plan is a **unification** of several earlier proposals.
7 The **merger** of Italy did not occur until the second half of the nineteenth century.
8 The company made its fortune by selling a popular **union** of coffee.
9 The proposed **federation** of the Liberal and Labour Parties in the election was cause for much ridicule.
10 As a result of the **compound** with the other company, Flax International became the largest in its field.

10 Reason and result

A Join the first part of the sentence in the left-hand column with the second part from the right-hand column, using an appropriate expression showing reason or result from the central column. In some cases, more than one of the expressions from the middle is possible.

1 The police asked him . . . . his . . .	. . . ensued . . .	. . . pass his exams.
2 He failed his exam . . .	. . . effects of . . .	. . . wake anyone.
3 A persistent cough . . .	. . . prompted him to . . .	. . . was unable to enrol for the
4 She started haranguing the crowd . . .	. . . on account of . . .	course.
5 He spent the whole weekend revising . . .	. . . as a consequence . . .	. . . upsetting me like that?
6 They came in quietly . . .	. . . affect . . .	. . . his lack of revision.
7 He refused to lend anyone money . . .	. . . owing to . . .	. . . starting a riot.
8 The bank manager refused to lend the	. . . on the grounds that . . .	. . . its low turnover and poor sales
company more money . . .	. . . so as not to . . .	history.
9 The school was forced to close . . .	. . . with the aim of . . .	. . . its action.
10 What were your . . .	. . . in order to . . .	. . . when the police officers on trial
11 What are the . . .	. . . consequences of . . .	were acquitted.
12 Stress and overwork can . . .	. . . motives in . . .	. . . a large earthquake?
13 The army attacked without considering the . . .	. . . due to . . .	. . . people rarely repay a loan.
14 He failed to send off his application form	. . . reason for . . .	. . . seek professional medical help.
and . . .		. . . different people in different ways.
15 Riots and street fighting . . .		. . . poor student attendance.
		. . . speeding through the town.

B Now complete these sentences with an appropriate expression from the central column of the table above.

1 Panic buying . . . . when the stock market crashed.
2 People often do things without considering the . . . . their actions.
3 The government raised the income tax rate . . . . curb inflation.
4 The government raised the income tax rate . . . . curbing inflation.
5 The government raised the income tax rate . . . . the rapidly rising rate of inflation.
6 When questioned, many racists cannot give a logical . . . . their attitudes towards other racial groups.
7 The soaring crime rate alarmed the police superintendent and . . . . adopt a zero-tolerance policing policy.
8 He was arrested . . . . he was a danger to others and himself.
9 The family was forced to economise . . . . go heavily into debt.
10 The fumes from motor traffic . . . . people in many different ways.

11 Generalisations and specifics

A   Match the sentences in the first list with an appropriate sentence in the second list. The *italic expressions* in the first list should have a similar meaning to the words or expressions in **bold** in the second list.

First list

1   *Small items of information* are very important in a curriculum vitae.
2   I need to have *precise information* about your new proposals.
3   The plan was unable to go ahead because of *a small important detail which is important in order to make something happen.*
4   He demanded to know the *small, precise and sometimes unimportant details.*
5   When you read a piece of text in the exam, you should read it quickly first to get the *general idea*.
6   Before you write an essay, you should plan it first and give *a broad description without giving much detail.*
7   *Odd features or details which make something different* make the world a more interesting place.
8   Saying that all seventeen-year-olds take drugs is a bit of a *general statement*.
9   Many cars have very similar *typical features*.
10 The huge rise in computer sales is a good *example* of the direction in which technology is heading.
11 *Normally,* most students sitting the exam manage to pass with a good grade.
12 The new library *shows a good example of* British architecture at its best.
13 Before you travel somewhere, it is important to *make a detailed list of* things that you need to take.
14 French fries with mayonnaise is a dish which is *an odd feature or detail* of Belgian cuisine.
15 The article *shows as an example* his views on the way the company should develop.

Second list

A   Please let me have the **specifics** as soon as possible.
B   It's very frustrating when a minor **technicality** puts a stop to your plans.
C   In the same way, kimchii is a concoction of cabbage, chilli and garlic which is **peculiar to** Korea.
D   You should include full **details** of your past experience.
E   Once you have an **outline**, you will discover that your work is easier to organise.
F   We must be careful not to make too many **generalisations**.
G   **Itemise** everything in order of importance, beginning with your passport and visa.
H   As far as he was concerned, the **minutiae** could not be overlooked.
I   Most manufacturers are aware that these **characteristics** are what help sell their product.
J   It also provides us with an accurate **illustration** of the advances we have made in the last twenty years.

K   It **illustrates** his preference for increased automation.

L   Once you have the **gist**, it should be easier to understand it.

M   It **exemplifies** the style that is becoming increasingly popular with town planners.

N   **In general**, the average result is a B or C.

O   For example, it is a **peculiarity** of the British system that judges and lawyers wear wigs.

B   Write a list of the words and expressions in bold above. Put them into two groups based on whether they are talking about general things or specific things. Try to give examples of each word in a sentence of your own.

Don't forget to keep a record of the words and expressions that you have learnt, review your notes from time to time and try to use new vocabulary items whenever possible.

A Rearrange the letters in **bold** to form words which are used to focus attention on something. They all end with the letters *-ly*. Write the words in the grid underneath. If you do it correctly, you will find another word used to focus attention in the bold vertical box.

1 They reduced pollution **pislmy** by banning cars from the city centre during the rush hour.
2 The strange weather at the moment is **gaerlly** due to El Niño.
3 We're examining **iilmprary** the financial aspects of the case.
4 People **ilnamy** go on holiday in the summer.
5 The library is **veceslxuily** for the use of students and staff.
6 It's a **ilaptarrculy** difficult problem which we hope to resolve as soon as possible.
7 The advertisement is **elcifipcsaly** aimed at people over 50.
8 Some western countries, **otbanly** Canada and the United States, have a very high standard of living.
9 The staff are **stomly** women of about twenty.
10 Our trip to Poland was **rpeluy** an educational visit.
11 My home town is famous **hfiecly** for its large number of schools and colleges.

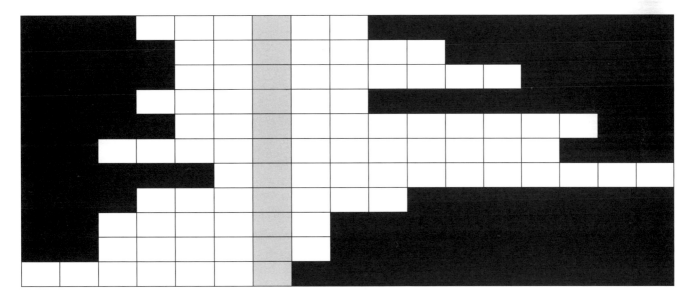

The word in the bold vertical strip fits into this sentence:

The company trades . . . . in the Far East.

B Divide the words above into two groups, one group being the words which mean *only* or *solely*, and one group being the words which mean *in most cases, normally* or *the main reason for something*.

Only or solely	In most cases, normally or the main reason for something

A The words in **bold** in the following sentences are all used to talk about opinion and belief. However, the words are *grammatically incorrect* (for example, a noun has been used instead of an adjective, or a verb has been used instead of a noun, etc.) or sometimes a noun has been used which has the wrong meaning. Put the words into their correct form.

1 In my **opinionated**, technology is moving too quickly.
2 As far as I am **concerning**, happiness is more important than money.
3 Scientists are **convincingly** that human degradation of the environment is causing thousands of species to become extinct.
4 The government are **regardless** the Third World debt as a major problem to global economic development.
5 Hundreds of people called the television station to register their **disapprove** of the presenter's behaviour.
6 She **maintenance** that most young people would rather work than go to school.
7 Do you **reckoning** that there will be an election in the next two years?
8 We strongly **suspicion** that the proposal to develop the computer facilities will not go ahead.
9 I **doubtful** that the new government will keep all its promises.
10 Do you **disapproval** of smoking?
11 I take strong **except** to people coming late or cancelling appointments at short notice.
12 A lot of people are **fanatic** about sport in general and football in particular.
13 British health inspectors are **obsession** about cleanliness in restaurant kitchens.
14 After years of struggle, the **moderations** have gained control of the party.
15 He has very **conservatism** views and disapproves of change.
16 The government are **commitment** to the struggle to end institutional racism in the police force.
17 She was **dedication** to her family and would do anything to protect them.
18 They come from a strongly **tradition** family who still believe in arranged marriages.

B Put these nouns and adjectives, which describe people's beliefs, under the most appropriate heading in the table. Can you think of any other words or expressions that you could add?

- opinionated   • a republican   • pragmatic   • a Muslim   • an intellectual
- a revolutionary   • tolerant   • a moralist   • narrow minded   • bigoted
- open-minded   • a vegan   • left-wing   • right-wing   • a socialist
- a royalist   • a Buddhist   • a conservative   • a liberal   • a communist
- a vegetarian   • dogmatic   • moral   • a fascist   • religious   • a Hindu
- middle-of-the-road   • an anarchist   • a stoic

Political beliefs	Personal convictions and philosophies

14 Stopping something

A For each of the examples 1–15, choose an appropriate verb from the box which best fits the description and can be used in the sample sentence.

> • back out   • sever   • quash   • suppress   • deter   • dissuade   • give up
> • cancel   • remove   • turn down   • put an end to   • delete   • repeal
> • rescind   • deny

1 To cut out part of a document, a computer file, etc.
   To stop your hard disk becoming too full, you should . . . . any unwanted programmes.

2 To officially end a law so that it is no longer valid.
   The new government Bill seeks to . . . . the existing legislation.

3 To discourage someone from doing something.
   The threat of severe punishment didn't . . . . the thieves from striking again.

4 To persuade someone not to do something.
   The college tries to . . . . students from entering exams which are not suitable for them.

5 To annul or cancel a contract or agreement.
   The committee decided to . . . . its earlier resolution on the use of its premises.

6 To limit something, such as a person's freedom.
   The military government attempted to . . . . the democracy movement by arresting its leaders.

7 To end something suddenly and finally.
   The Cornucopian government decided to . . . . relations with Utopia.

8 To refuse something which is offered.
   You should never . . . . a good job when it's offered to you.

9 To decide not to support or be part of a project or activity after you have agreed to do so.
   We decided to . . . . when we discovered the company was in financial difficulty.

10 To state that something is not correct.
   Before his trial, his lawyer advised him to . . . . embezzling company funds.

11 To stop something which has been planned.
   There is no refund if you . . . . your holiday less than three weeks before the date of the departure.

12 To make a judging or ruling no longer valid.
   He applied for a judicial review to . . . . the verdict.

13 To stop doing something that you have done for quite a long time.
   You should . . . . smoking if you want to feel healthier.

14 To stop something which has been going on for a long time.
   They agreed to . . . . their long-standing dispute.

15 To take something away.
   I would be grateful if you would . . . . my name from your mailing list.

15 Objects and actions

A The words in the box describe the actions of the things in 1–37. Match each action with the thing it describes.

> • evaporate   • explode   • change   • melt   • fade   • bounce   • crumble
> • trickle   • rise   • sink   • ring   • contract   • crack   • escape
> • stretch   • wobble   • congeal   • burn   • spill   • smoulder   • erupt
> • spin   • revolve   • set   • flow   • slide   • rotate   • spread   • erode
> • meander   • turn   • subside   • freeze   • grow   • expand   • vibrate
> • float

1 The planet Earth moving round on its axis.
2 A washing machine in its final stage of a wash.
3 The moon moving around the Earth.
4 The CD-ROM tray on a computer base unit.
5 A house slowly sinking into soft ground.
6 Water slowly being converted into vapour.
7 Cooking fat becoming solid on an unwashed plate.
8 Traffic moving smoothly along a motorway.
9 Water changing from a liquid to a solid because of the cold.
10 Glass changing from a solid to a liquid in very high heat.
11 A loose wheel on a car.
12 Gas coming out of a faulty valve.
13 A rubber ball hitting the ground and going back into the air.
14 Loose windows in a window frame when a large vehicle passes nearby.
15 The population of a town becoming bigger.
16 A T-shirt which has been washed so often it has lost its colour.
17 The sun coming up in the morning.
18 The sun going down in the evening.
19 A wheel on a slow-moving train.
20 Traffic lights going from red to amber to green.
21 Cliffs being slowly destroyed by the sea.
22 Documents being laid out on a table.
23 A wide river winding through the countryside.
24 The sun turning people on a beach bright red.
25 An incense stick in the entrance to a temple.
26 A lump of dry earth being rubbed between somebody's fingers.
27 Cold metal as it gets hotter.
28 Hot metal as it gets cooler.
29 A piece of elastic being pulled so that it becomes longer.

30 A window being hit by a stone so that a long, thin break is formed.

31 Coffee falling out of a cup by mistake.

32 A bomb suddenly blowing up.

33 An alarm clock suddenly going off.

34 A boat going to the bottom of a river.

35 Dead fish lying on the surface of a polluted lake.

36 A volcano throwing out lava and ash.

37 Orders for a new product arriving at a company very slowly.

B Several of the words in the box above can have more than one meaning. Use your dictionary to check which ones, then complete these sentences below with an appropriate word. You may need to change the form of some of the words.

1 The queues for the embassy were so long they . . . . all the way down the street.

2 'What do you think you're doing?' he . . . . angrily.

3 The government decided that the best economic course would be to let the dollar . . . .

4 Prices have been . . . . steadily all year.

5 The light from the torch began to . . . . as the batteries ran out.

6 The twig . . . . loudly as he stood on it.

7 After the rainstorms passed, the floodwaters gradually . . . .

8 The discussion . . . . around the problem of student accommodation.

9 The doctor . . . . his broken arm.

10 The car . . . . out of control on the icy road.

16 Likes and dislikes

A Look at the words and expressions in the box and decide if they have a positive connotation (for example, they tell us that somebody *likes* something) or a negative connotation (for example, they tell us that somebody *dislikes* something).

- loathe   • yearn for   • passionate about   • fond of   • captivated by
- fancy   • keen on   • look forward to   • dread   • long for   • appeal to
- detest   • cannot stand   • repel   • attracted to   • fascinated by
- tempted by   • disgust   • revolt   • cannot bear

B Now look at these pairs of sentences. Sometimes, both sentences are correct, sometimes one of them is wrong (for example, the construction is wrong) or it does not sound natural. Decide which ones.

1 A. It was well-known that he was loathed by the other teachers.
   B. It was well-known that the other teachers loathed him.

2 A. Sometimes I yearn for some time on my own.
   B. Sometimes some time on my own is yearned for.

3 A. Sport is passionate about by a lot of people.
   B. A lot of people are passionate about sport.

4 A. Animals are quite fond of by British people.
   B. British people are quite fond of animals.

5 A. The first time I visited Venice, I was captivated by the city.
   B. The first time I visited Venice, the city captivated me.

6 A. Going to the cinema tonight is fancied by me.
   B. I fancy going to the cinema tonight.

7 A. From a young age, the idea of travelling was keen on me.
   B. From a young age I was keen on the idea of travelling.

8 A. I look forward to hearing from you soon.
   B. To hearing from you soon I look forward.

9 A. It is a well-known fact that students dread exams.
   B. It is a well-known fact that exams are dreaded by students.

10 A. Most children long for the long summer holiday to arrive.
    B. The long summer holiday is longed for by most children.

11 A. His sense of humour is appealed to by watching other people suffer.
    B. Watching other people suffer appeals to his sense of humour.

12 A. Racism is really detested by me.
    B. I really detest racism.

13 A. A lot of people cannot stand the long British winters.
    B. The long British winters cannot be stood by a lot of people.

14 A. The idea of living in a cold country repels me.
    B. I am repelled by the idea of living in a cold country.

Likes and dislikes

15 A. She was attracted to the tall, handsome man who had helped her.
   B. The tall, handsome man who had helped her attracted her.

16 A. I have always been fascinated by information technology.
   B. Information technology has always fascinated me.

17 A. Were you tempted by his offer of a job in Australia?
   B. Did his offer of a job in Australia tempt you?

18 A. His mannerisms and habits disgusted me.
   B. I was disgusted by his mannerisms and habits.

19 A. Bigoted, arrogant people revolt me.
   B. I am revolted by bigoted, arrogant people.

20 A. Getting up early in the morning cannot be born by me.
   B. One thing I cannot bear is getting up early in the morning.

17 Time

A Use the time clauses in the boxes to complete the sentences. Pay particular attention to the words that come before or after the time clause.

Part 1: One action or situation occurring before another action or situation

• prior to	• previously	• earlier	• formerly	• precede	• by the time

1 . . . . the advent of the Industrial Revolution, pollution was virtually unheard of.
2 . . . . the army had restored order, the city had been almost completely devastated.
3 . . . . known as Burma, the republic of Myanmar is undergoing a slow and painful political transformation.
4 A sudden drop in temperature will usually . . . . a blizzard.
5 It was my first trip on an aeroplane. . . . . I'd always gone by train.
6 The Prime Minister made a speech praising charity organisations working in Mozambique. . . . . that day he had promised massive economic aid to stricken areas.

Part 2: One action or situation occurring at the same time as another action

• while/as/just as	• during/throughout	• at that very moment
• in the meantime/meanwhile		

1 . . . . the minister was making his speech, thousands of demonstrators took to the streets.
2 . . . . the speech they jeered and shouted slogans.
3 The minister continued speaking. . . . . the police were ordered onto the streets.
4 He finished the speech with a word of praise for the police. . . . . the sun came out and shone down on the assembled crowd of happy supporters.

Part 3: One action or situation occurring after another action or situation

---

> • **afterwards**   • **as soon as/once/the minute that**   • **following**

1 . . . . the earthquake, emergency organisations around the world swung into action.
2 . . . . the stock market collapsed, there was panic buying on an unprecedented scale.
3 The Klondike gold rush lasted from 1896 to 1910. . . . . the area became practically deserted overnight.

B Look at these words and expressions and decide if we usually use them to talk about (1) the past, (2) the past leading to the present, (3) the present or (4) the future. Try to write a sentence for each one.

> • **for the next few weeks**   • **as things stand**   • **ever since**   • **in medieval times**
> • **nowadays**   • **from now on**   • **back in the 1990s**   • **over the past six weeks**
> • **over the coming weeks and months**   • **in another five years' time**   • **one day**
> • **in those days**   • **a few decades ago**   • **lately**   • **at this moment in time**
> • **at the turn of the century**   • **in my childhood/youth**   • **at this point in history**
> • **by the end of this year**   • **for the foreseeable future**   • **for the past few months**
> • **last century**   • **these days**   • **from 1996 to 1998**   • **sooner or later**

Don't forget to keep a record of the words and expressions that you have learnt, review your notes from time to time and try to use new vocabulary items whenever possible.

18 Obligation and option

A Look at sentences 1–10 and decide if the explanation which follows each one is true or false. Use the words and expressions in **bold** to help you decide.

1 During the exam, a pencil and eraser are **required**.
The people organising the exam will provide you with a pencil and an eraser.

2 Parents can be made **liable for** their children's debts.
Parents may be legally responsible for the money their children owe.

3 He was **obliged** to pay back the money that he had won.
He had the choice whether or not to pay back the money that he had won.

4 Students doing holiday jobs are **exempt** from paying income tax.
Students doing holiday jobs pay a smaller amount of income tax than other people.

5 The United Nations voted to impose **mandatory** sanctions on the country.
The United Nations imposed legally-binding sanctions which had to be obeyed by everyone, without exception.

6 The doctors **forced** him to stop smoking.
The doctors asked him to stop smoking.

7 It was an emergency and she pressed the red button; there was **no alternative**.
There was nothing else she could do; she had to set off the alarm by pressing the red button.

8 Classes on Wednesday afternoons are **optional**.
It is necessary to attend classes on Wednesday afternoons.

9 It is **compulsory** to wear a crash helmet on a motorcycle.
It is your choice whether or not to wear a crash helmet when you ride a motorcycle.

10 The museum is asking visitors for a **voluntary** donation of £2.
You don't need to pay £2 to visit the museum.

B Complete these sentences with an appropriate word or expression from the exercise above. In some cases, more than one answer may be possible.

1 Visitors to the country are . . . . to declare any excess tobacco or alcohol imports to the customs officer.

2 I'm afraid I have . . . . but to resign from the committee.

3 If you are caught speeding, you will be . . . . the payment of the fine.

4 Attendance at all classes is . . . . , otherwise you may not get a certificate at the end of the course.

5 Many retired people do . . . . work in their local community.

6 In some countries, there is a . . . . death sentence for all drug traffickers.

7 For visitors to Britain from outside the European Union, a visa may be . . . .

8 He said he was innocent, but the police . . . . him to confess.

9 Most new cars come with . . . . air-conditioning.

10 Children's clothes are . . . . from VAT.

Don't forget to keep a record of the words and expressions that you have learnt, review your notes from time to time and try to use new vocabulary items whenever possible.

19 Success and failure

A Match the first part of each sentence in the left-hand column with its second part in the right-hand column using an appropriate word from the central column. These words should collocate with the **bold** words in the right-hand column. In most cases, it is possible to use the words in the central column with more than one sentence.

Success

1	The two warring countries managed to . . .	. . . secure . . .	. . . his **ambitions** of being promoted to marketing manager.
2	During his first year as President he managed to . . .	. . . accomplish . . .	. . . my **aims** of doing well at school and then going to university.
3	The company couldn't afford to move to new premises but were able to . . .	. . . attain . . .	. . . an **agreement** for a new lease.
4	He worked hard at his job and was soon able to . . .	. . . achieve . . .	. . . its **targets** – those of free education and healthcare – within eight years.
5	The country badly needed to increase its overall standard of living and attempted to . . .	. . . fulfil . . .	. . . his **obligations** to his current employer.
6	After four years of hard work, the motor racing team managed to . . .	. . . realise . . .	. . . their **goal** of becoming millionaires.
7	He desperately wanted to start a new job, but first of all he had to . . .	. . . reach . . .	. . . their **dreams** of winning the Monaco Grand Prix.
8	Many people want to be rich but few . . .		. . . **a lot more** than his predecessor had in the previous five.
9	I have a lot of plans, and one of them is to . . .		. . . a **compromise** over the terms for peace.

B Complete these sentences with an appropriate word or expression from A, B or C.

Failure

1 The People's Foundation Party decided to . . . . its plans to establish a coalition government with the Democratic Liberal Party.
   A. abate   **B. abandon**   **C. abhor**

2 Peace talks between the two countries . . . ., with neither side able to agree on terms.
   A. collapsed   **B. collaborated**   **C. collared**

3 Progress in the talks . . . . when the inevitable impasse was reached.
   A. faulted   **B. faltered**   **C. fondled**

4 Our planned visit to the Czech Republic . . . . because we were unable to get the visas.
   A. fell over   **B. fell down**   **C. fell through**

5 The company . . . . with debts of over £1 million.
   A. faulted   **B. folded**   **C. foiled**

6 Their plans to impose stricter import quotas . . . . when the European Bank declared their actions illegal.
   A. mistook   **B. mislead**   **C. misfired**

20 Ownership, giving, lending and borrowing

Nouns

A Complete sentences 1–13 with an appropriate word from the box. In some cases, more than one answer may be possible.

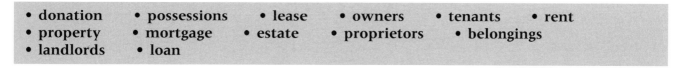

• donation • possessions • lease • owners • tenants • rent
• property • mortgage • estate • proprietors • belongings
• landlords • loan

1 The law ensures that . . . . respect the privacy of the people who live in their houses.
2 . . . . of restaurants across the country protested at the new government tax that was put on food.
3 Private car . . . . were hit the hardest when tax on petrol was increased.
4 The price of commercial . . . . has almost doubled in the last four years.
5 When the recession hit, he was forced to sell his 250-acre . . . .
6 Many families lost all their . . . . when the river flooded.
7 Put your . . . . in the locker and give the key to the receptionist.
8 We will need to relinquish the offices when the . . . . runs out at the end of the year.
9 They applied to the World Bank for a . . . . to help pay off their balance of payments deficit.
10 A lot of people lost their homes when the interest rate rose so much they were unable to pay off their . . . .
11 The . . . . complained to the council that the house they were living in was overrun with vermin.
12 The law does little to protect families who are thrown out of their homes because they are unable to pay the . . . .
13 Everybody is being asked to make a . . . . to help the victims of the disaster.

Verbs

B The words in **bold** have been put into the wrong sentences. Decide which sentences they should belong in. In some cases, more than one answer is possible.

1 Banks will refuse to **rent** money to anyone without sufficient collateral.
2 If you want to **contribute** a room in the centre of the city, you should be prepared to pay a lot of money.
3 The best way to see the country is to **provide** a car from an agency for a couple of weeks.
4 Companies **allocate** from banks to finance their business.
5 It is not only the wealthy who **provide for** money to charities.

6 It is our responsibility to **leave** our parents when they get old.
7 The government will tax you heavily for any money that your relatives may **lend** for you in their will.
8 Local councils will **borrow** free accommodation to the most needy on a first-come, first-served basis.
9 Charities such as the Red Crescent **hire** free medical aid to areas hit by disasters.

21 Around the world

A. Choose the correct geo-political word in A, B or C to complete each of these sentences.

1 Japan, Korea and the Philippines are all in the . . . .
   A. Near East   **B. Middle East**   **C. Far East**

2 The South Pole is situated in the . . . .
   A. Arctic   **B. Antarctic**   **C. Antarctica**

3 New Zealand is part of . . . .
   A. Australia   **B. Australasia**   **C. Austria**

4 Bangladesh is part of . . . .
   A. the Indian Subcontinent   **B. India**   **C. Indiana**

5 Nicaragua is a country in . . . .
   A. North America   **B. South America**   **C. Central America**

6 Argentina, Brazil, Colombia, Panama and Honduras all form part of . . . .
   A. Latin America   **B. Spanish America**   **C. South America**

7 Apartheid was abolished in . . . . in the 1990s.
   A. southern Africa   **B. North Africa**   **C. South Africa**

8 The United Kingdom and the Republic of Ireland form a group of islands known as . . . .
   A. Great Britain   **B. England**   **C. The British Isles**

9 The United Kingdom and the Republic of Ireland form part of . . . .
   A. Continental Europe   **B. Mainland Europe**   **C. Europe**

10 Kuwait, Oman and the United Arab Emirates form part of what is known as . . . .
   A. the West Indies   **B. the Gulf States**   **C. the European Union**

11 Norway, Sweden, Finland and Denmark are known collectively as . . . .
   A. the Baltic Republics **B. the Caribbean**   **C. Scandinavia**

B Change each country/area below into the nationality and/or language spoken of the people who come from that place (For example: Britain = Brit*ish*). Write each word in the appropriate space in the table. Be careful, because usually we add or remove letters to/from the name of the country before we add the ending.

• **Greece**	• **Portugal**	• **Ireland**	• **Belgium**	• **Finland**	• **England**
• **Wales**	• **Scotland**	• **Holland**	• **Lebanon**	• **Malaysia**	• **Norway**
• **Sweden**	• **Thailand**	• **Peru**	• **Bangladesh**	• **Israel**	• **Japan**
• **Russia**	• **Iran**	• **Burma**	• **America**	• **Canada**	• **Spain**	• **Turkey**
• **Kuwait**	• **Switzerland**	• **Arabia**	• **Denmark**	• **Yemen**	• **Iraq**
• **Australia**	• **Malta**	• **Philippines**	• **Poland**		

-ese (e.g. China = Chinese)	-(i)an (e.g. Brazil = Brazilian)	-ish (e.g. Britain = British)	-i (e.g. Pakistan = Pakistani)	-ic (e.g. Iceland = Icelandic)	Others (e.g. France = French)

C   A quick quiz. Answer these questions.

1   What do we call a variety of language spoken in a particular area? Is it an accent, a dialect or an idiom?

2   What is **your** *mother tongue*?

3   What do we call a person who is able to speak (a) two languages and (b) three or more languages fluently?

4   With regard to your country, what is (a) the name of the continent in which it is located, (b) the main language spoken and (c) the nationality of the people.

22 Groups

A Put these words into the table based on the group of things they usually refer to.

- batch   - huddle   - heap/pile   - company   - stack   - team   - litter
- swarm   - flock   - platoon   - bundle   - herd   - throng   - gang
- crowd   - bunch   - set   - pack   - staff   - group   - crew   - cast
- shoal/school

People in general	People working together	Animals	Objects

B Complete these sentences using one of the words from the above task. In some cases, more than one answer is possible.

1 After the election, the huge . . . . danced in the street.

2 The refugees sat in a small, tight . . . . underneath some trees.

3 The first prize was a . . . . of cheap saucepans.

4 The school is closed because the . . . . are on strike.

5 The theatre . . . . benefited from a government grant.

6 Following an outbreak of BSE, a . . . . of cows has been destroyed.

7 The company processed a . . . . of orders.

8 A . . . . of football fans wandered around the street breaking shop windows.

9 Half the . . . . of the film were nominated for Oscars.

10 They threw the weapons in a . . . . on the ground.

11 A small . . . . of people petitioned the Prime Minister outside his house.

12 The . . . . of fish that had been caught were deemed inedible owing to pollution in the water.

13 We were all surprised when our dog gave birth to a . . . . of puppies.

14 Cabin . . . . on aircraft are drilled in safety procedure.

15 As winter approaches, the . . . . of geese fly south to warmer climes.

16 Half the football . . . . were sent off in disgrace.

17 The stars had difficulty making their way through the . . . . of people outside the cinema.

18 A . . . . of soldiers from the Third Infantry have been charged with human rights abuses.

19 The immigrant arrived clutching nothing but a . . . . of personal possessions.

20 A . . . . of flowers is always an acceptable gift if you visit someone.

21 We were unable to open the door because a . . . . of boxes was blocking it.

22 The women fell on the surprised burglar like a . . . . of wild dogs.

23 The harvest was destroyed by a huge . . . . of insects.

C The following words all refer to groups of people meeting for a specific purpose. Match the words with their definitions in the list below.

- **delegation**   - **tribunal**   - **symposium**   - **seminar**   - **lecture**   - **tutorial**

A students listening to a talk on a particular subject

B a group of representatives (for example, of a union) who want to explain something to someone

C a student or small group of students who attend a teaching session

D a meeting organised to discuss a specialised subject

E a small group of university students discussing a subject with a teacher

F a specialist court outside the main judicial system which examines special problems and makes judgements

23 Shape and features

A (Shape) Match the words below with the picture that best represents each word.

1 pyramid	2 cube	3 crescent	4 spiral	5 cone	6 sphere
7 rectangle	8 triangle	9 square	10 circle	11 cylinder	12 oval

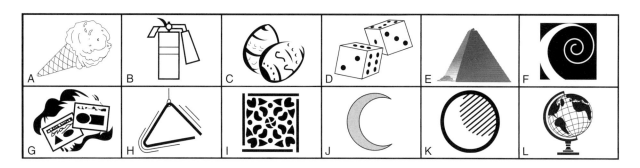

B (Shape) Look at the following list of words and decide what the correct adjective form is, A, B or C.

1	Sphere	A. spherous	B. spherical	C. spherocous
2	Cube	A. cubed	B. cubous	C. cubal
3	Cone	A. conacular	B. conous	C. conical
4	Rectangle	A. rectanglous	B. rectanglis	C. rectangular
5	Triangle	A. triangular	B. trianglous	C. triangled
6	Circle	A. circled	B. circulous	C. circular
7	Square	A. square	B. squaret	C. squarous
8	Cylinder	A. cylindrous	B. cylindal	C. cylindrical

C (Features) Match the descriptions on the left with the objects, geographical features, etc., on the right.

1	a sharp edge with jagged teeth	A	a country road in very poor condition
2	steep, with a pointed peak	B	somebody's hair
3	rolling, with undulating wheat fields	C	a very old tree
4	curved, with a smooth surface	D	a knife
5	flat, with words and dotted lines	E	a slow-moving river
6	wavy, with blonde hi-lights	F	a mountain
7	meandering, with a calm surface	G	a banana
8	winding and bumpy, with deep potholes	H	agricultural countryside
9	hollow, with rough bark	I	an application form

24 Size, quantity and dimension

A Look at the following list and decide whether we are talking about something *big* (in terms of size, quantity or dimension) or something *small*.

1 a **minute** amount of dust . . . .
2 a **minuscule** piece of cloth . . . .
3 an **enormous** book. . . . .
4 a **mammoth** job. . . . .
5 a **huge** waste of time. . . . .
6 a **vast** room. . . . .
7 a **gigantic** wave. . . . .
8 a **tiny** car. . . . .
9 a **monumental** error. . . . .
10 a **colossal** statue. . . . .
11 **plenty** of food. . . . .
12 **dozens** of times. . . . .
13 a **narrow** alleyway. . . . .
14 a **giant** building . . . .
15 a **gargantuan** meal. . . . .
16 a **wide** avenue. . . . .
17 a **broad** river. . . . .
18 a **tall** man. . . . .
19 a **high** mountain. . . . .
20 a **deep** lake. . . . .
21 a **shallow** pool. . . . .
22 a **long-distance** journey. . . . .
23 a **vast** crowd of supporters. . . . .
24 **tons** of work. . . . .
25 a **great deal of** time. . . . .

B Now complete these sentences using one of the expressions above. In some cases, more than one answer is possible.

1 Before you embark on . . . ., it is essential that you are well-prepared.
2 We spent . . . . working on the plans for the new library.
3 I've told you . . . . not to smoke in here.
4 . . . . must have blown into the camera and scratched the film.
5 Villages along the coast were destroyed when . . . . caused by the earthquake swept houses into the sea.
6 It was . . . . going there; he didn't even turn up.

7 One of the Roman emperor Nero's greatest excesses was to build . . . . of himself in the city centre.

8 Despite the poor harvest, there was . . . . for the whole population.

9 . . . . called the Thames separates the city of London from the suburbs to the south.

10 . . . . gathered to see their favourite football team.

11 We ate . . . . and then lay down to rest.

12 It was . . . . and his voice echoed around the walls.

13 We have . . . . to do in the next few days, so I suggest we start as soon as possible.

14 Loch Ness is . . . . in the Highlands of Scotland.

15 The only evidence was . . . . which was stuck on a branch of one of the trees in the garden.

16 'Sumo' is . . . . containing almost 1,000 pictures by the controversial photographer Helmut Newton.

17 He had . . . . to do, so took the phone off the hook, made himself some coffee and sat down at his desk.

18 The Matterhorn, ... in Switzerland, has claimed the lives of many who have tried to climb it.

19 He made . . . . in his calculations and had to start all over again.

20 The manufacturers have built . . . . which is ideal for getting around the city.

21 The NEC in Birmingham is . . . . which is used for concerts and exhibitions.

22 The main feature of the town is a . . . . lined with shops and cafés.

23 I could see the key glittering at the bottom of . . . .

24 Legend spoke of . . . . dressed in gold, known as El Dorado.

25 . . . . ran along the side of the house to a garden at the rear.

25 Emphasis and misunderstanding

A (Emphasis) Match the sentences on the left with an appropriate sentence on the right.

1	The minister's **emphasis** on the word 'peace' was noticeable.	A	The government will have to sit up and take note of what these **important** people have to say.
2	Our guide **accentuated** the importance of remaining calm if there was trouble.	B	She **emphasised** the fact that panicking would only make matters worse.
3	Our teacher explained that it was **crucially important** to pace ourselves while revising for the exam.	C	The leader **gave prominence to** the need to create better job opportunities.
4	At the People's Party conference, the **accent** was on youth unemployment.	D	We consider progress in this field to be **extremely important.**
5	**Prominent** trade unionists have called for a boycott of imported goods.	E	He **put great stress** on the maxim that 'All work and no play makes Jack a dull boy'.
6	It is **of crucial importance** that we make more use of technology if we are to make progress.	F	He **stressed** again and again the importance of an established détente.

B (Emphasis) Now complete these sentences with an expression in **bold** from the above exercise. In some cases, more than one answer may be possible.

1 Some medical treatments do very little to help the patient. In fact, in some cases, they only . . . . the pain.

2 The revolution began when a . . . . member of the ruling party was assassinated.

3 At the meeting of the Students' Council, the . . . . was on better standards of accommodation.

4 She . . . . the need to be fully prepared for all eventualities while travelling.

5 The Minister of Transport . . . . on the need for an integrated transport policy.

6 It is . . . . that we try to improve relations between our countries.

7 She banged the table for . . . . as she spoke.

C (Misunderstanding) Complete sentences 1–9 with an appropriate word or expression from the box. In some cases, more than one answer is possible.

- **mix-up**   - **obscure**   - **impression**   - **distorted**   - **misapprehension**
- **mistaken**   - **confusion**   - **assumed**   - **confused**

1 She was . . . . by the journalist's questions.
2 There were scenes of . . . . at the airport when the snowstorm stopped all the flights.
3 We nearly didn't catch our flight because of a . . . . over the tickets.
4 There are several . . . . points in his letter. It's not very clear.
5 He . . . . the meaning of my speech, creating the false impression that I was a racist.
6 He was under the . . . . that socialism and communism were the same thing.
7 The jury . . . . , wrongly, that he was innocent.
8 They were . . . . in the belief that the refugees were in the country for economic rather than political reasons.
9 The press were under the . . . . that the Prime Minister was about to resign.

26 Changes

A Look at these sentences and decide if the statement which follows each one is *true* or *false*. Use the words and expressions in **bold** to help you decide.

1 The population of the country has trebled in the last 25 years.
   *There has been a **dramatic increase** in the number of people living in the country.*

2 Unemployment has dropped by about 2% every year for the last six years.
   *There has been a **steady decrease** in the number of people out of work.*

3 The government has spent a lot of money improving roads around the country.
   *There has been a **deterioration** in the national road system.*

4 The number of exam passes achieved by the school's pupils has risen by almost 50%.
   *There has been a **decline** in the number of exam passes.*

5 American travellers abroad have discovered that they can buy more foreign currency with their dollar.
   *There has been a **weakening** of the dollar.*

6 It is now much easier to import goods into the country than it was a few years ago.
   *There has been a **tightening up** of border controls.*

7 We're increasing our stocks of coal before the winter begins.
   *We're **running down** our stocks of coal.*

8 Prices have gone up by about 4% every year since 1998.
   *There has been a **constant rise** in the rate of inflation.*

9 The pass rate for the exam was 3% lower this year than it was last year.
   *There has been a **sharp fall** in the pass rate.*

10 The alliance are going to reduce the number of conventional weapons in their armed forces.
    *The alliance are going to **build up** the number of weapons they have.*

11 Deflation has adversely affected industries around the country.
    *There has been a **growth** in industrial activity.*

12 The rules are much stricter now than they were before.
    *There has been a **relaxation** of the rules.*

13 Last year, 12% of the population worked in industry and 10% worked in agriculture. This year, 14% of the population work in industry and 8% work in agriculture.
    *There has been a **narrowing of the gap** between those working in different sectors of the economy.*

14 Some management roles in the company will not exist this time next year.
    *Some management roles are going to be **phased out**.*

15 More people are shopping at large supermarkets rather than small village shops.
    *There has been an **upward trend** in the number of people shopping in small village shops.*

16 Her English is clearly better now than it was when she first arrived.
    *There has been **marked progress** in her English.*

17 People live in better houses, drive nicer cars and eat higher-quality food than they did twenty years ago.
    *There has been a **general improvement** in the standard of living.*

18 Our company has opened factories in France, Germany and Italy in the last five years.
    *Our company has witnessed considerable **expansion** in the last five years.*

19 The government will spend less on the National Health Service next year.
*There are going to be **cuts** in healthcare spending next year.*

20 British people nowadays want to see more of the world.
*British people nowadays want to **narrow** their horizons.*

B Check your answers, then use some of the words and expressions in **bold** above and in the answer key to write some sentences about your country.

27 Opposites

Replace the words in **bold** in these sentences with a word from the box which has an opposite meaning.

Verbs

> • withdrew • fell • rewarded • loosened • refused (to let) • set
> • denied • deteriorated • abandoned • forbade • lowered
> • demolished • retreated • simplified • defended • rejected

1 They **accepted** the offer of a ceasefire.
2 He **admitted** telling lies in his original statement.
3 The army slowly **advanced**, leaving a trail of devastation in its path.
4 They **agreed** to meet to discuss the future of the organisation.
5 The minister **attacked** his party's policies in a speech in Parliament.
6 The apartments blocks they **built** were the ugliest in the city.
7 He **complicated** matters by rewriting the original proposal.
8 They **continued** their plans to assassinate the king when he opened the parliament.
9 He **deposited** £7,000 – half his college fees for the forthcoming year.
10 Relations between the two countries have **improved** considerably in the last year.
11 He **permitted** us to present our petition directly to the President.
12 The members of the commune were **punished** for their part in the revolution.
13 He **raised** the overall standards of the company within two months of his appointment.
14 As soon as the sun **rose**, the demonstrators began to appear on the streets.
15 Prices **rose** sharply in the first three months of the financial year.
16 As soon as he had **tightened** the knots, he pushed the boat out.

Adjectives

> • scarce • easy • approximate • dim • compulsory • delicate
> • innocent • detrimental • reluctant • crude • even • clear
> • graceful • clear • flexible

1 The meaning of his words was very **ambiguous**.
2 According to his colleagues, he's a very **awkward** person to deal with.
3 When she first started dancing, she was very **awkward**.
4 His policies were **beneficial** to the economy as a whole.
5 We need **exact** figures before we embark on a new venture.

6 The jury decided he was **guilty** of the crime.

7 Add up all the **odd** numbers between 1 and 20 to get a result.

8 Despite the weather, supplies of food after the harvest were **plentiful**.

9 The laws protecting the green belt around the city are very **rigid**.

10 There is a **slight** difference in the way the company is run these days compared with a few years ago.

11 The device is very **sophisticated** and should only be operated by someone who is familiar with it.

12 The spices used in the production of some international dishes have a very **strong** flavour.

13 The **strong** light from the torch picked out details on the walls of the cave.

14 Attendance at afternoon classes should be **voluntary**.

15 A lot of students are **willing** to attend classes on Saturday morning.

> Don't forget to keep a record of the words and expressions that you have learnt, review your notes from time to time and try to use new vocabulary items whenever possible.

28 Addition, equation and conclusion

This module will help you to review more of the important words that we use to join ideas in an essay, a verbal presentation or sometimes in everyday speech (*see also* Module 1: Condition and Module 8: Contrast and comparison).

A Put the following words and expressions into their correct place in the table depending on their function.

- to sum up briefly   • along with   • it can be concluded that   • also
- likewise   • similarly   • besides   • to conclude   • too   • in addition
- in brief   • in the same way   • thus   • what's more   • furthermore
- moreover   • along with   • to summarise   • as well as   • therefore
- correspondingly

Addition (For example: and)	Equation (For example: equally)	Conclusion (For example: in conclusion)

B   Complete these sentences with one of the words or expressions from above. In most cases, more than one answer is possible.

1   Tourism brings much needed money to developing countries. . . . . , it provides employment for the local population.

2   . . . . bringing much needed money to developing countries, tourism provides employment for the local population.

3   Tourists should respect the local environment. . . . . they should respect the local customs.

4   . . . . industrial waste, pollution from car fumes is poisoning the environment.

5   In order to travel, you need a passport. . . . . , you might need a visa, immunisation jabs and written permission to visit certain areas.

6   Drugs are banned in Britain – . . . . . weapons such as guns and knives.

7   All power corrupts. . . . . , absolute power corrupts absolutely.

8   You shouldn't smoke, drink, take drugs or eat unhealthy food. . . . . , you should live a more healthy lifestyle.

9   The ozone layer is becoming depleted, the air in the cities is becoming too dirty to breathe and our seas and rivers are no longer safe to swim in. . . . . pollution is slowly destroying the planet.

10 Your grades have been very poor all years. . . . . you need to work really hard if you want to pass your exams next month.

29 Task commands

Look at the list of tasks in the first list. In particular, look at the words in **bold**, which are telling the writer/speaker what he/she must do. Match these words with a suitable definition of the task command in the second list. Two of these definitions can be used more than once.

1 **Account for** the increased use of technology in modern society.
2 **Analyse** the effects of climactic change around the world.
3 **Assess** the improvements you have made in your English since you started using this book.
4 **Compare** the lifestyles of young people in Britain and young people in your country.
5 **Define** the word 'hope'.
6 **Demonstrate** the different features of this computer.
7 **Discuss** the advantages and disadvantages of growing up in a single-parent family.
8 **Elaborate** on your feelings about capital punishment.
9 **Estimate** the costs of setting up a website for the company.
10 **Evaluate** how useful our class visit to the Bank of England was.
11 **Examine** the causes of global warming.
12 **Explain** the sudden interest in old-fashioned toys such as yo-yos.
13 **Identify** the person who attacked you.
14 **Illustrate** the problems the National Health Service is currently facing.
15 **Justify** your reasons for refusing to help me.
16 **Outline** the history of the motor car in the last fifty years.
17 **Predict** the changes that we are going to see in information technology in the next ten years.
18 **Suggest** ways in which you can become a more efficient student.
19 **Summarise** your feelings towards a united Europe.
20 **Trace** the development of nuclear technology from its earliest days.

A Describe what you think can be done in order to achieve something.
B Tell in advance what you think will happen.
C Explain, with real examples, why something has happened or is happening.
D Give a brief history of something, in the order in which it happened.
E Give the meaning of something.
F Talk about something with someone else, or write about it from different viewpoints.
G Calculate (but not exactly) the value or cost of something.
H Give a broad description of something without giving too much detail.
I Explain something closely and scientifically.
J Write or talk about the different aspects (e.g., causes, results) of something.
K Explain something in more detail than you did previously.
L Look at two things side by side to see how they are similar or different.
M Explain something in a few main points, without giving too much detail.

N   Say why something has happened.

O   Show or prove that something is right or good.

P   Show how something works, usually by physically operating it so that the other person knows what it does and how it works.

Q   Give a physical description of somebody.

R   Calculate the value of something.

30 Confusing words and false friends

Confusing words

Confusing words are two or more words which

- have a similar meaning to each other but are used in a different way

or

- are related to the same topic, but have a different meaning

or

- look similar, but have a different meaning.

False friends

False friends are words in English which have a similar-looking word in another language but which have a different meaning.

Complete the following sentences with the appropriate word.

1 **action/activity**
   The police took immediate . . . . when they realised the situation was getting out of hand.
   Economic . . . . stagnated as the recession took hold.

2 **advice/advise**
   Can you . . . . me on the best course of action to take?
   He offered me some excellent . . . .

3 **affect/effect**
   Cuts in spending will have a serious . . . . on the National Health Service.
   The strike will seriously . . . . train services.

4 **appreciable/appreciative**
   There is an . . . . difference between manslaughter and murder.
   She was very . . . . of our efforts to help.

5 **assumption/presumption**
   They raised taxes on the . . . . that it would help control spending.
   It's sheer . . . . for the government to suggest things have improved since they came to power.

6 **avoid/prevent**
   Rapid government reforms managed to . . . . a revolution taking place.
   He's always trying to . . . . taking a decision if he can help it.

7 **beside/besides**
   The office is just . . . . the railway station.
   . . . . their regular daytime job, many people do extra work in the evening.

8 **briefly/shortly**

. . . . before the conflict began, the army pulled down the border posts.

The minister spoke . . . . about the need for political reform.

9 **channel/canal**

The television . . . . received a formal complaint about the programme.

The Suez . . . . was built in the second half of the nineteenth century.

10 **conscientious/conscious**

Most people are . . . . of the need to protect the environment.

. . . . workers should be rewarded for their hard work.

11 **continual/continuous**

A . . . . trade embargo has badly affected the economic infrastructure.

The computer has given us . . . . problems ever since we installed it.

12 **control/inspect**

Environmental health officers regularly . . . . kitchens and other food preparation areas.

The government plans to . . . . the price of meat to make sure it doesn't go up too much.

13 **criticism(s)/objection(s)**

They didn't raise any . . . . when we insisted on inspecting the figures.

The government's plan was met with severe . . . .

14 **damage/injury/harm**

It was a severe . . . . which needed immediate hospital treatment.

A lot of . . . . was caused to buildings along the coast during the storm.

There's no . . . . in taking a break from your job now and then.

15 **discover/invent**

When did he . . . . the telephone?

Did Alexander Fleming . . . . penicillin?

16 **during/for/while**

Shops were closed . . . . the duration of the conflict.

. . . . the transition from a dictatorship to democracy, the country experienced severe strikes and riots.

The bomb went off . . . . the President was making his speech.

17 **however/moreover**

The plan was good in theory. . . . . , in practice it was extremely difficult to implement.

The plan was excellent. . . . . , it was clear from the beginning that it was going to be a success.

18 **inconsiderate/inconsiderable**

An . . . . amount of money was wasted.

. . . . behaviour makes life unpleasant for everybody.

19 **intolerable/intolerant**

I consider his behaviour to be quite . . . .

The government is . . . . of other political parties.

20 **job/work**

Everybody has the right to a decent . . . . with good pay.

Following the recession, many people are still looking for . . . .

21 **lay(s)/lie(s)**

The city of Quito . . . . near the equator.

The manager made it clear he intended to . . . . down some strict rules.

22 **look at/watch**

We must . . . . the situation in Lugumba carefully, and be prepared to act if violence flares again.

We need to . . . . the problem carefully and decide if there is anything we can do about it.

23 **permission/permit**

I'm afraid we can't . . . . photography in here.

They received . . . . to attend the sessions as long as they didn't interrupt.

24 **possibility/chance**

There is always the . . . . that the government will reverse its decision.

If we act now, we have a good . . . . of finding a cure for the disease.

25 **practice/practise**

It's important to . . . . your English whenever possible.

You need more . . . . before you take the exam.

26 **priceless/worthless**

. . . . paintings by artists like Van Gogh should not be in the hands of private collectors.

As inflation spiralled out of control, paper money suddenly became . . . .

27 **principal(s)/principle(s)**

Many people refuse to eat meat on . . . .

The . . . . of the college is an ardent non-smoker.

The country's . . . . products are paper and wood.

Not many people are familiar with the . . . . of nuclear physics.

28 **process/procession**

The . . . . made its way down the avenue.

Applying for a visa can be a long and frustrating . . . .

29 **raise/rise**

As prices . . . ., demand usually drops.

In response to the current oil shortage, most airlines plan to . . . . their fares.

30 **respectable/respectful**

The delegates listened in . . . . silence as the chairman spoke.

They want to bring up their children in an area which is considered to be . . . .

31 **treat/cure**

Hospitals are so understaffed that they find it almost impossible to . . . . patients with minor injuries.

They were unable to . . . . the disease, and hundreds died as a result.

31 Useful interview expressions

Below you will see some common expressions that you might find useful in the IELTS speaking test. Put each expression into the correct box according to the function of that expression.

1 May I think about that for a moment?
2 In short, . . .
3 What I'm trying to say is . . .
4 to sum up, . . .
5 What are your views on . . . ?
6 Would you mind repeating that?
7 How can I put this?
8 In other words . . .
9 Sorry to butt in . . .
10 Well, as a matter of fact . . .
11 I'm not so sure about that
12 Pardon?
13 I can't help thinking the same
14 What are your feelings about . . . ?
15 So in conclusion, . . .
16 I see things rather differently myself
17 True enough
18 That's right
19 I don't entirely agree with you

20 Perhaps I should make that clearer by saying . . .
21 How can I best say this?
22 Could you repeat what you said?
23 I couldn't agree more
24 Actually . . .
25 To put it another way . . .
26 That's just what I was thinking
27 In brief, . . .
28 Could I just say that . . .
29 Well, my own opinion is that . . .
30 That's my view exactly
31 To summarise, . . .
32 What was that?
33 I must take issue with you on that
34 Let me get this right
35 Sorry to interrupt, but. . . .
36 I'm afraid I didn't catch that
37 What's your opinion?

Agreeing with somebody
Example: Yes, I agree.

Disagreeing with somebody
Example: I'm afraid I disagree.

Interrupting

Example: Excuse me for interrupting.

Asking for clarification or repetition

Example: I'm sorry?

Asking somebody for their opinion

Example: What do you think about . . . ?

Saying something in another way

Example: What I mean is . . .

Giving yourself time to think

Example: (in response to a question) Let me see.

Summing up

Example: So basically . . .

32 Phrasal verbs

Phrasal verbs (a verb and a preposition/prepositions combined to form a new expression) are a large and very important area of English vocabulary which many students ignore. There are a lot of them, and many phrasal verbs can have more than one meaning.

Below, on the left, you will see a list of many of the verbs which are used to make phrasal verbs. On the right you will see the prepositions which can work with these verbs to form phrasal verbs. Use a dictionary to find out which verb/preposition combinations are possible and complete the table.

You should try to build up a bank of the phrasal verbs which you are unfamiliar with and which you think are important. On page 108, there is a record sheet which you can photocopy as many times as you like, make a note of phrasal verbs on, and add to your files.

*Don't forget that some phrasal verbs use more than one preposition (for example, **We ran up against** some problems).*

Verb	Prepositions which can be added to form phrasal verbs	Preposition
Come		
Cut		about
Get		
Give		across
Go		after
Look		along
Make		aside
Pick		
Put		at
Run		away
Set		back
Take		
Turn		behind
Break		

Call		by
Carry		do
Count		down
End		for
Face		forward
Fall		in
Hang		into
Hold		off
Keep		on
Let		out
Pull		over
Show		round
Sort		through
Split		
Wear		to
Work		up
		without

Phrasal verb record sheet

Main verb:

Phrasal verb	Definition	Sample sentence(s)

Continue onto a new page if you need to add more phrasal verbs to your list.
You may photocopy this page.

33 Spelling: commonly misspelled words

A Each paragraph in this information leaflet contains one spelling mistake. Identify the mistake and correct it in each case. When you have finished, check the key and explanatory notes at the back of this book. Then do exercise B below.

Welcome to St. Clarissa's!
1 Welcome to St. Clarissa's School of English. We hope you have an enjoyable stay with us. We suggest that you pay attention to the following advise if you want to make the most of your time here.
2 Attend all your lessons and do all your homework so that you can acheive your aims.
3 Make the most of your free time to aquire new learning skills which you can use when you return to your country and continue to study English.
4 Don't forget to make optimum use of the college sports facilities, including the gym and swiming pool.
5 Take care of your personal belongings at all times. It is not unusual for thiefs to steal things from the classrooms.
6 Students hopeing to continue their studies at a British university should talk to the Educational Services officer.
7 Your happyness here is very important to us. Speak to your personal tutor if you have any problems.

B When you have checked the answers to the above exercise, identify and correct the spelling mistakes in these sentences.

1 I respect the party's acknowledgment of defeat in the election.
2 It is argueable whether travel is faster now than it was fifty years ago.
3 Very few people are currently benefitting from social security.
4 Many South-East Asian states are doing a lot of busness with European countries.
5 The government's anti-smoking campain is having little effect.
6 Cancelations will be accepted until a week before departure.
7 Weather conditions can be very changable in maritime climates.
8 There is no point condeming the council for their lack of action.
9 Consientious students do not always get the best results.
10 The hieght of the bridge is only four metres.
11 In some countries, financial problems are too large to be managable.
12 His speech decieved millions.
13 Hundreds of lifes are being lost daily due to careless drivers.
14 Earthquake survivers often remain in shock for several days.
15 It is essential to practice daily if you want to become a good musician.

C Not all English words have rules to help you remember how they are spelt. In many cases, you must learn each individual word. Look at the sentences below. Each one contains a word which is often spelt incorrectly. Choose the correct spelling, A, B or C, for each sentence.

1 The former president was sentenced in his . . . .
A. absence   **B. absance**   **C. abscence**

2 The first step to becoming a good photographer is to buy the correct . . . .
A. accesories   **B. accessories**   **C. acessories**

3 Visitors have difficulty finding . . . . during the summer.
A. acommodation   **B. accommodation**   **C. accomodation**

4 City planners can sometimes be very . . . . in their approach to traffic calming.
A. aggressive   **B. aggresive**   **C. agressive**

5 The managing director made an important . . . . to his staff.
A. anouncement   **B. announcment**   **C. announcement**

6 The college offers a course in commercial . . . .
A. correspondance   **B. corespondence**   **C. correspondence**

7 Between 1997 and 2001, a . . . . drop will be seen in the market.
A. defenite   **B. definate**   **C. definite**

8 The government openly . . . . of the current judicial system.
A. dissaproves   **B. disapproves**   **C. diseproves**

9 Governments need to . . . . with the current judicial system.
A. liase   **B. leaise**   **C. liaise**

10 A lot of people do not have the . . . . qualifications for the job.
A. necesary   **B. neccesary**   **C. necessary**

11 A car is a . . . . if you live in the country.
A. necessity   **B. neccesity**   **C. necesity**

34 Education

Task 1: Look at the sentences below and fill in the gaps using the appropriate word from A, B or C.

1 He didn't get a good grade the first time he did his IELTS exam, so decided to . . . . it.
   A. resit   **B. remake**   **C. repair**

2 People who attend university later in life are often called . . . . students.
   A. aged   **B. mature**   **C. old**

3 Although she had left school and was working, she went to evening classes at the local College of . . . . Education.
   A. Upper   **B. Further**   **C. Higher**

4 After he left school, he decided to go on to . . . . education and applied for a place at Edinburgh University.
   A. further   **B. upper**   **C. higher**

5 He received a local government . . . . to help him pay for his course.
   A. fee   **B. fare**   **C. grant**

6 Education helps us to acquire knowledge and learn new . . . .
   A. skills   **B. powers**   **C. abilities**

7 Although she already had a first degree from university, she decided that she wanted to work towards a . . . . degree later in life.
   A. further   **B. senior**   **C. higher**

8 We should make the best of every . . . . to learn.
   A. chance   **B. opportunity**   **C. availability**

9 Nowadays, ... education is promoted a lot in schools.
   A. body   **B. health**   **C. vitality**

10 A large number of parents are dissatisfied with the . . . . education system, and put their children into private schools instead.
   A. government   **B. national**   **C. state**

11 Because so many students find exams stressful, some colleges offer a system of . . . . assessment instead.
   A. continual   **B. continuous**   **C. ongoing**

12 He has read a lot of books and . . . . a lot of knowledge.
   A. acquired   **B. won**   **C. achieved**

Task 2: Complete sentences 1–11 with a suitable word or expression from the box.

• primary	• numeracy	• graduate	• evening class	• course	• discipline
• literacy	• day release	• kindergarten	• enrol	• secondary	• skills
• pass	• correspondence	• qualifications	• degree		

1 When Michael was three, he started going to a . . . .

2 At the age of five, he entered . . . . education.

3 He learned basic . . . . such as . . . . and . . . .

4 After he turned eleven he began to attend . . . . school.

5 Although he was lazy and lacked sufficient . . . . , he was able to . . . . his exams.

6 When he was eighteen he found a college which offered a . . . . in Art and Design.

7 He was able to . . . . for the course a few days before his nineteenth birthday.

8 He worked hard and three years later was able to . . . . with a . . . . in Art and Design.

9 After that he followed a . . . . course in photography from a college in the USA using the Internet.

10 The . . . . he gained impressed an advertising company he wanted to work for.

11 Although he is now working, he has decided to attend an . . . . after work, although he was disappointed that his boss didn't offer him . . . .

Task 3: Now read this essay and complete the gaps with one of the words or expressions from Tasks 1 and 2. You may need to change the form of some of the words.

'You are never too old to learn'. Do you agree with this statement?

Education is a long process that not only provides us with basic (1) . . . . such as (2) . . . . and (3) . . . . , but is also essential in shaping our future lives. From the moment we enter (4) . . . . as small children, and as we progress through (5) . . . . and (6) . . . . education, we are laying the foundations for the life ahead of us. We must (7) . . . . ourselves to work hard so that we can (8) . . . . exams and gain the (9) . . . . we will need to secure a good job. We must also (10) . . . . valuable life skills so that we can fit in and work with those around us. And of course (11) . . . . education helps us to understand how we can stay fit and healthy.

For most people, this process ends when they are in their mid-to-late teens. For others, however, it is the beginning of a lifetime of learning. After they finish school, many progress to (12) . . . . education where they will learn more useful skills such as computer literacy or basic business management. Others will (13) . . . . on a programme of (14) . . . . education at a university where, with hard work, they will have the opportunity to (15) . . . . after three or four years with a well-earned (16) . . . . After that, they may work for a while before opting to study for a (17) . . . . degree – an MA, for example, or a PhD. Alternatively, they may choose to attend an (18) . . . . after work or, if they have a sympathetic employer, obtain (19) . . . . so that they can study during the week. And if they live a long way from a college or university, they might follow a (20) . . . . course using mail and the Internet. In fact, it is largely due to the proliferation of computers that many people, who have not been near a school for many years, have started to study again and can proudly class themselves as (21) . . . . students.

We live in a fascinating and constantly changing world, and we must continually learn and acquire new knowledge if we are to adapt and keep up with changing events. Our schooldays are just the beginning of this process, and we should make the best of every (22) . . . . to develop ourselves, whether we are eighteen or eighty. You are, indeed, never too old to learn.

35 The media

Task 1: Match the words and expressions in Box A with a suitable definition in Box B.

Task 2: Complete this extract from a television interview with an appropriate word or expression from the box.

Interviewer: Welcome to today's programme. Today we will be discussing the (1) . . . . , and asking the question: Should we allow newspapers and television channels to print or say whatever they like? In the studio I have television personality Timothy Blake and (2) . . . . Robert Poubelle, multi-millionaire owner of the *Daily Views* newspaper. Timothy, let's start with you.

T.B.: Thank you. In my opinion, it's time the government imposed stricter (3) . . . . of the press in order to prevent (4) . . . . journalists and reporters from making money by (5) . . . . people. I have often accused Mr Poubelle's organisation of (6) . . . . – nowadays I can't even sunbathe in my garden without being photographed by his hordes of (7) . . . . They're like vultures. And everything they print about me is lies, complete rubbish.

Interviewer: But isn't it true that the media provides us with valuable (8) . . . . and (9) . . . . , and censorship would deprive us of much of this? Robert?

R.P.: Of course. Mr. Blake's accusations are unfounded, as are the accusations of (10) . . . . we have received, but I can safely say that my journalists never pay people money to create stories. We are simply reporting the truth. Of course, if Mr. Blake wants to sue us for (11) . . . ., he is very welcome to try. But he would be depriving our (12) . . . . – all eight million of them – of the things they want. . . . .

T.B.: You're talking rubbish, as usual, like the pathetic (13) . . . . you own and use to fill your pockets with dirty money.

R.P.: Now look here, mate . . .

Task 3: Now read this essay and complete the gaps with one of the words or expressions from Tasks 1 and 2. You may need to change the form of some of the words.

'The media plays a valuable role in keeping us informed and entertained. However, many people believe it has too much power and freedom.' Discuss your views on this, giving examples and presenting a balanced argument both in favour of, and against, the power and freedom of the media.

Barely a hundred years ago, if we wanted to stay informed about what was going on in the world, we had to rely on word of mouth or, at best, newspapers. But because communication technology was very basic, the news we received was often days or weeks old.

We still have newspapers, of course, but they have changed almost beyond recognition. Whether we choose to read the (1) . . . ., with their quality (2) . . . . of news and other (3) . . . . by top (4) . . . . and articles by acclaimed (5) . . . ., or if we prefer the popular (6) . . . ., with their lively gossip and colourful stories, we are exposed to a wealth of information barely conceivable at the beginning of the last century.

We also have television and radio. News (7) . . . . let us know about world events practically as they happen, while sitcoms, chat shows and documentaries, etc. keep us entertained and informed. And there is also the (8) . . . ., where we can access information from millions of (9) . . . . around the world which we can then (10) . . . . onto our own computers.

However, these forms of (11) . . . . and (12) . . . . (or 'infotainment' as they are now sometimes collectively called) have their negative side. Famous personalities frequently accuse the (13) . . . . (and sometimes even respectable papers) of (14) . . . . by the (15) . . . . who are determined to get a story at any cost. Newspapers are often accused of (16) . . . . by angry politicians who dislike reading lies about themselves, and there are frequent accusations of (17) . . . ., with (18) . . . . reporters paying people to create stories for their newspapers or television programmes. Of course, it is not just the papers which are to blame. Sex and violence are increasing on the television. Undesirable people fill the (19) . . . . with equally undesirable material which can be accessed by anyone with a home computer. And the fear of (20) . . . . prevents many from (21) . . . . to the Internet.

Many argue that the government should impose stricter (22) . . . . to prevent such things happening. But others argue that (23) . . . . is the keystone of a free country. Personally, I take the view that while the media may occasionally abuse its position of power, the benefits greatly outweigh the disadvantages. Our lives would be much emptier without the wealth of information available to us today, and we are better people as a result.

Task 1: How would you generally feel, happy ☺ or unhappy ☹, if you were in the following situations? Use the words in **bold** to help you decide.

1 The company you work for is well-known for its **job security**. ☺ ☹
2 You were suddenly **made redundant**. ☺ ☹
3 You received a **promotion**. ☺ ☹
4 You were given an **increment**. ☺ ☹
5 You worked **unsociable hours**. ☺ ☹
6 You had a **steady job**. ☺ ☹
7 You had **adverse working conditions**. ☺ ☹
8 You suddenly found yourself **unemployed**. ☺ ☹
9 You took time off work because of **repetitive strain injury**. ☺ ☹
10 The office where you work has **sick building syndrome**. ☺ ☹
11 You receive regular **perks** as part of your job. ☺ ☹
12 Somebody called you a **workaholic**. ☺ ☹
13 Your company doesn't give you many **incentives**. ☺ ☹
14 Your boss announces that there is going to be some **downsizing** of the workforce. ☺ ☹
15 Your work didn't offer much **job satisfaction**. ☺ ☹
16 Your company has a generous **incentive scheme**. ☺ ☹
17 You receive a **commission** for the work you have done. ☺ ☹
18 You receive support from a **union**. ☺ ☹
19 You were under **stress**. ☺ ☹
20 You were forced to **resign**. ☺ ☹
21 You received a **cut** in your **salary**. ☺ ☹
22 Your company gave you **sickness benefit**. ☺ ☹
23 You found your job very **demanding**. ☺ ☹

Task 2: Match sentences 1–6 below with one of the sentences A–F. Use the words in **bold** to help you.

1 Samantha is the assistant manager of a bank and she works from 8.30 to 5.30 every day.
2 Tracy works on the production line of a factory which makes cars. She uses a machine to spray paint onto the finished car parts.
3 Jane works for herself. She is a photographer. She works every day for about eight or nine hours.
4 Jeanette is a cleaner for a company in Birmingham, but she only works there for about three or four hours a day.
5 Claire has a powerful job in the personnel office of a large multinational company. She is responsible for employing new people and getting rid of those that the company doesn't want to employ anymore.
6 Marie works in the finance department of an international college in Oxford.

A She is a **semi-skilled blue-collar worker** in a **manufacturing industry**.

B She is **self-employed** and works **full-time**. She likes to describe herself as **freelance**.

C She is responsible for **hiring and firing**.

D She calculates the **wages, salaries, pension contributions** and **medical insurance contributions** of all the staff.

E She is a **full-time white-collar worker** in a **service industry**.

F She is an **unskilled part-time employee**.

Task 3: Now read this essay and complete the gaps with one of the words or expressions from Tasks 1 and 2. You may need to change the form of some of the words.

'Some people live to work, and others work to live. In most cases, this depends on the job they have and the conditions under which they are employed. In your opinion, what are the elements that make a job worthwhile?'

In answering this question, I would like to look first at the elements that combine to make a job *un*desirable. By avoiding such factors, potential (1) . . . . are more likely to find a job that is more worthwhile, and by doing so, hope to achieve happiness in their work.

First of all, it doesn't matter if you are an (2) . . . . worker cleaning the floor, a (3) . . . . (4) . . . . worker on a production line in one of the (5) . . . . , or a (6) . . . . worker in a bank, shop or one of the other (7) . . . . : if you lack (8) . . . . , with the knowledge that you might lose your job at any time, you will never feel happy. Everybody would like a (9) . . . . in which he or she is guaranteed work. Nowadays, however, companies have a high turnover of staff, (10) . . . . new staff and (11) . . . . others on a weekly basis. Such companies are not popular with their workers.

The same can be said of a job in which you are put under a lot of (12) . . . . and worry, a job which is so (13) . . . . that it takes over your life, a job where you work (14) . . . . and so never get to see your family or friends, or a physical job in which you do the same thing every day and end up with the industrial disease that is always in the papers nowadays – (15) . . . .

With all these negative factors, it would be difficult to believe that there are any elements that make a job worthwhile. Money is, of course, the prime motivator, and everybody wants a good (16) . . . . But of course that is not all. The chance of (17) . . . . , of being given a better position in a company, is a motivating factor. Likewise, (18) . . . . such as a free lunch or a company car, an (19) . . . . scheme to make you work hard such as a regular (20) . . . . above the rate of inflation, (21) . . . . in case you fall ill and a company (22) . . . . scheme so that you have some money when you retire all combine to make a job worthwhile.

Unfortunately, it is not always easy to find all of these. There is, however, an alternative. Forget the office and the factory floor and become (23) . . . . and work for yourself. Your future may not be secure, but at least you will be happy.

Don't forget to keep a record of the words and expressions that you have learnt, review your notes from time to time and try to use new vocabulary items whenever possible.

37 Money and finance

Task 1: Use a dictionary to find the differences between the words and expressions in **bold** in the following groups.

1 make **a profit** and make **a loss**
2 **extravagant** and **frugal/economical**
3 a **current account** and a **deposit account**
4 a **loan** and a **mortgage**
5 to **deposit** money and to **withdraw** money
6 a **wage** and a **salary**
7 **broke** and **bankrupt**
8 **shares, stocks,** and **dividends**
9 **income tax** and **excise duty**
10 to **credit** and to **debit**
11 a **bank** and a **building society**
12 a **discount** and a **refund**
13 something which was a **bargain,** something which was **overpriced** and something which was **exorbitant**
14 **worthless** and **priceless**
15 **save** money and **invest** money
16 **inflation** and **deflation**
17 **income** and **expenditure**
18 to **lend** and to **borrow**

Task 2: Match the sentences in column A with the sentences in column B. Use the words in **bold** to help you.

	Column A		Column B
1	The managing director believes the company should start producing pocket computers.	A	I'm really looking forward to spending my **pension**.
2	I always put my money in a building society and not in a bank.	B	The **cost of living** seems to go up every day.
3	I can't afford to buy a new car right now. I don't have enough money.	C	Of course, it's always so difficult to **economise**.
4	I find Christmas a very expensive time.	D	Shops all over the country are making huge **reductions** on just about everything.
5	I came into a lot of money recently when my uncle died.	E	I always seem to run up a huge **overdraft** at the bank.
6	Look at this cheque that came in the post this morning from the Inland Revenue.	F	Of course, the potential global **market** for them is enormous.
7	I've been spending too much recently.	G	Fortunately I receive **unemployment benefit**.
8	In my country, there are a lot of very poor people and only a few rich ones.	H	There is a very uneven **distribution of wealth**.
9	I lost my job last month.	I	The **interest** they pay me is much higher.
10	I retire next month.	J	It's the first time I've **inherited** something.
11	Prices are rising quickly everywhere.	K	It seems to be some kind of tax **rebate**.
12	The January sales start tomorrow.	L	Maybe I should consider getting one **on credit**.

Task 3: Now read this passage and complete the gaps with one of the words or expressions from Tasks 1 and 2. You may need to change the form of some of the words.

'Financial advice from a father to a son'

In the play 'Hamlet' by William Shakespeare, a father gives his son some financial advice. 'Neither a borrower nor a lender be', he says. He is trying to tell his son that he should never (1) . . . . money from anyone because it will make it difficult for him to manage his finances. Likewise he should never give a financial (2) . . . . to a friend because he will probably never see the money again, and will probably lose his friend as well.

The play was written over four hundred years ago, but today many parents would give similar advice to their children. Imagine the conversation they would have now:

Son: Right dad, I'm off to university now.

Father: All right son, but let me give you some sound financial advice before you go.

Son: Oh come on dad . . .

Father: Now listen, this is important. The first thing you should do is to make sure you balance your (3) . . . . – the money you receive from me – and your (4) . . . . – the money you spend. If you spend too much, you will end up with an (5) . . . . at the bank. Don't expect me to pay it for you.

Son: But it's so difficult. Things are so expensive, and the (6) . . . . goes up all the time. (7) . . . . is running at about 10%.

Father: I know, but you should try to (8) . . . . Avoid expensive shops and restaurants. Also, put your money in a good (9) . . . . They offer a much higher rate of (10) . . . . than banks. Also, avoid buying things (11) . . . .

Son: Why?

Father: Because shops charge you an (12) . . . . amount of money to buy things over a period of time. It's much better to (13) . . . . a little bit of money each week so that when you see something you want, you can buy it outright. Try to wait for the sales, when shops offer huge (14) . . . . and you can pick up a (15) . . . . And try to get a (16) . . . .

Son: How do I do that?

Father: Easy. When you buy something, ask the shop if they'll lower the price by, say, 10%. Next, when you eventually get a job and are earning a good salary, try to (17) . . . . the money in a good company. Buy (18) . . . . in government organisations or (19) . . . . in private companies.

Son: OK dad, I've heard enough.

Father: One final piece of advice, son.

Son: What's that dad?

Father: To thine own self be true.

Son: You what?

Task 1: Look at the sentences 1–12 and rearrange the letters in **bold** to make a word connected with politics. (The first and last letters of each word are <u>underlined</u>. A dictionary definition is included to help you.) Then put the words into the grid below. If you do it correctly, you will find a word in the bold vertical strip which means 'rule of a country by one person'.

1 We live in a **meyoadcrc**. (a country governed by freely elected representatives of the people)
2 Scotland is aiming for **ndnpniedceee** in the next few years. (freedom)
3 A **aidtdenac** for the Labour Party called at our house last week. (a person who is standing for election)
4 The military junta abolished the constitution and set up a **ioaialrttan** régime. (having total power and not allowing any opposition or personal freedom)
5 An **huiatoitaarrn** government is not necessarily a bad thing. (controlling people strictly)
6 The Prime Minister has appointed a group of **octthraecns** to run the government. (a person with particular skills brought in to run a country or an organisation)
7 The Conservative Party lost the election and is now in **opsionotip**. (the party or group which opposes the government)
8 France is a **picubrel**, with a president and prime minister. (a system of government which is governed by elected representatives headed by an elected or nominated president)
9 Governments often impose strict economic **ontincsas** on countries which abuse their power. (restrictions on trade with a country in order to try to influence its political development)
10 The American Congress is formed of the **eoHus** of Representatives and the Senate. (part of a parliament)
11 Her socialist **oildgyoe** led her to join the party. (a theory of life based not on religious belief, but on political or economic philosophy)
12 **liarPatmen** has passed a law forbidding the sale of cigarettes to children. (a group of elected representatives who vote the laws of a country)

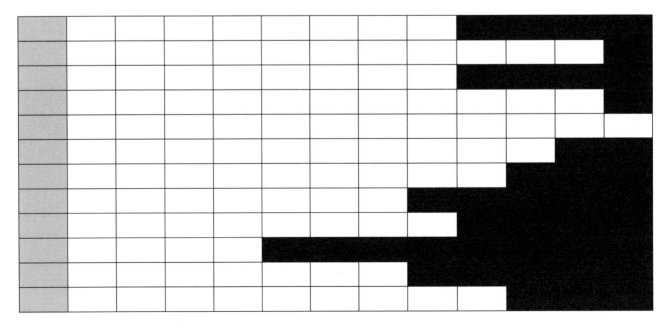

Task 2: Look at these sentences and decide if they are **true** or **false**. Use a dictionary to help you.

1 A **monarchy** is a system of government with an elected king or queen.
2 A **politician** is a person who works for the king or queen.
3 A **statesman** or **stateswoman** is an important religious leader or representative of a country.
4 A **cabinet** is a committee formed of the most important members of a government.
5 A **president** is the head of a republic.
6 A **ministry** is a person who works for the government.
7 A **constituency** is an area of a country which elects a Member of Parliament.
8 A **policy** is a government which is controlled by the police.
9 A **referendum** is the process of choosing by voting.
10 An **election** is a vote where all the people of a country are asked to vote on a single question.

Task 3: Now look at this extract from a current affairs radio programme and complete the gaps with one of the words or expressions from Tasks 1 and 2. In some cases, more than one answer may be possible. You may need to change the form of some of the words.

Good evening, and welcome to today's edition of 'Today in Government'

There were angry scenes in both (1) . . . . of Parliament today following an unprecedented walkout by the Prime Minister and other members of his (2) . . . . during a speech by the leader of the (3) . . . . Criticising their (4) . . . . on law and order, the Prime Minister called his opposite number a 'strict (5) . . . . who wants to take away the freedom of the individual and turn the country from a freedom-loving (6) . . . . to a (7) . . . . run by one man.'

It's almost time for the people of Britain to vote again and it is now only one month until the (8) . . . . All over the country, (9) . . . . from all the major parties are knocking on doors asking people to vote for them. We conducted a recent survey to find out who people will be voting for. Surprisingly, many support the Workers' Union Party for their policy of turning the country from a (10) . . . . to a (11) . . . . : a lot of people support the idea of getting rid of the Queen in favour of an elected president.

Members of Parliament have called for a (12) . . . . so that the people of Britain can decide whether or not the country joins the 'One Europe' organisation. This follows a survey in the town of Woolhampstead, the Prime Minister's own (13) . . . .

The Department of Education was accused by the press today of employing too many (14) . . . . Chris Smith, editor of the *Daily News*, defended his attack. 'It's no good having a department full of computer experts if they are unable to run our schools properly,' he said.

Michael Yates, a senior statesman for Britain at the European Commission, has called for EU member states to impose strict economic (15) . . . . on the government of Boland. This follows alleged human rights abuses on tribesmen in the north of the country who are demanding (16) . . . . Their leader, Asagai Walumbe, called on countries around the world to help them in their struggle for freedom.

39 The environment

Task 1: Match the first part of each sentence in the left-hand column with its second part in the right-hand column. Use the words in **bold** to help you. Check that each sentence you put together is grammatically correct.

1	Some modern agricultural methods have been heavily criticised, . . .	A	. . . in many countries **poaching** is considered more serious than drug smuggling.
2	If you wear a fur coat in public, . . .	B	. . . and **rare breeds** parks are very popular with many.
3	It is illegal to kill pandas, tigers . . .	C	. . . in **wildlife management**.
4	If we don't do more to protect pandas, . . .	D	. . . the government's **conservation programme** has been very successful.
5	A lot of British people are interested in unusual animals, . . .	E	. . . they'll soon be **extinct**.
6	National parks in Kenya are currently recruiting experts . . .	F	. . . with **battery farming** in particular receiving a lot of condemnation.
7	In an attempt to preserve forests around the country . . .	G	. . . it was fascinating to observe their **natural behaviour**.
8	We would like to carry out more scientific study into rainforests . . .	H	. . . on a successful panda **breeding** programme.
9	I don't like zoos because I think . . .	I	. . . keeping animals **in captivity** is cruel.
10	I saw a fascinating documentary about the way animals live in Venezuela and thought . . .	J	. . . or any other **endangered species**.
11	In order to increase the birth rate, the Chinese government has spent a lot of money . . .	K	. . . but it is often difficult to get people to fund the **research**.
12	Hunters have killed so many animals that . . .	L	. . . you risk coming under attack from **animal rights activists**.

Task 2: Replace the expressions in **bold** with a word or expression from the box which has the same meaning.

> • unleaded petrol   • fossil fuels   • recycle (things)   • organic
> • genetically modified   • greenhouse   • rain forest   • global warming
> • erosion   • contaminated   • environmentalists   • emissions
> • biodegradable packaging   • acid rain   • Green Belt   • ecosystem

1 In Britain, building is restricted or completely banned in the **area of farming land or woods and parks which surrounds a town**.

2 Many companies are developing **boxes, cartons and cans which can easily be decomposed by organisms such as bacteria, or by sunlight, sea, water, etc**.

3 The burning of some fuels creates **carbon dioxide, carbon monoxide, sulphur dioxide, methane and other** gases which rise into the atmosphere.

4 Farmers have cleared hectares of **thick wooded land in tropical regions where the precipitation is very high**.

5 Planting trees provides some protection from the **gradual wearing away** of soil.

6 We should all try to **process waste material so that it can be used again**.

7 These potatoes are **cultivated naturally, without using any chemical fertilisers and pesticides**.

8 This bread is made from wheat which has been **altered at a molecular level so as to change certain characteristics which can be inherited**.

9 More and more cars are built to use **fuel which has been made without lead additives**.

10 **Polluted precipitation which kills trees** falls a long distance away from the source of the pollution.

11 Human beings have had a devastating effect on the **living things, both large and small,** in many parts of the world.

12 The **gases and other substances** which come from factories using oil, coal and other **fuels which are the remains of plants and animals** can cause serious damage to the environment.

13 Don't drink that water! It's been **made dirty by something being added to it**.

14 Friends of the Earth, Greenpeace and other **people concerned with protecting the environment** are holding a forum in London next month.

15 **The heating up of the earth's atmosphere by pollution** is threatening life as we know it.

Task 3: Now look at this essay and complete the gaps with one of the words or expressions from Tasks 1 and 2. In some cases, more than one answer may be possible. You may need to change the form of some of the words.

'Environmental degradation is a major world problem. What causes this problem, and what can we do to prevent it?'

There is no doubt that the environment is in trouble. Factories burn (1) . . . . which produce (2) . . . . , and this kills trees. At the same time, (3) . . . . gases rise into the air and contribute to (4) . . . . , which threatens to melt the polar ice cap. Meanwhile farmers clear huge areas of (5) . . . . in places such as the Amazon to produce feeding land for cattle or produce wood for building. Rivers and oceans are so heavily (6) . . . . by industrial waste that it is no longer safe to go swimming. Cars pump out poisonous (7) . . . . which we all have to breathe in. (8) . . . . and overfishing are killing off millions of animals, including whales, elephants and other (9) . . . . In fact, all around us, all living things large and small which comprise our finely balanced (10) . . . . are being systematically destroyed by human greed and thoughtlessness.

There is a lot we can all do, however, to help prevent this. The easiest thing, of course, is to (11) . . . . waste material such as paper and glass so that we can use it again. We should also check that the things we buy from supermarkets are packaged in (12) . . . . packaging which decomposes easily. At the same time, we should make a conscious effort to avoid foods which are (13) . . . . (at least until someone proves that they are safe both for us and for the environment). If you are truly committed to protecting the environment, of course, you should only buy (14) . . . . fruit and vegetables, safe in the knowledge that they have been naturally cultivated. Finally, of course, we should buy a small car that uses (15) . . . . which is less harmful to the environment or, even better, make more use of public transport.

The serious (16) . . . . , however, do much more. They are aware of the global issues involved and will actively involve themselves in (17) . . . . by making sure our forests are kept safe for future generations. They will oppose activities which are harmful to animals, such as (18) . . . . And they will campaign to keep the (19) . . . . around our towns and cities free from new building.

We cannot all be as committed as them, but we can at least do our own little bit at grass roots level. We, as humans, have inherited the earth, but that doesn't mean we can do whatever we like with it.

40 Healthcare

Task 1: Match the sentence in the left-hand column with a sentence in the right-hand column. Use the words in **bold** to help you.

Problems

1	. . . Mrs Brady has suffered from terrible **rheumatism** for years.	A	Illnesses which affect the **circulation** of blood are particularly common with people who are overweight
2	. . . More women than men are affected by **arthritis**.	B	This is deposited on the walls of the **arteries** and can block them.
3	. . . Air conditioning units are often responsible for spreading **infections** around an office.	C	They can easily be spread from one person to another.
4	. . . **Cardiovascular disease** is becoming more common in Britain.	D	Pains or stiffness in the **joints** or **muscles** can be very difficult to live with.
5	. . . Too much exposure to the sun can cause skin **cancer**.	E	They don't get enough exercise.
6	. . . It is important not to eat too much food with a high **cholesterol** content.	F	Their **immune system** is not properly developed and can be easily hurt.
7	. . . Too many people these days live a **sedentary lifestyle**.	G	The painful **inflammation** of a joint may require **surgery**.
8	. . . People in positions of responsibility often have **stress-related** illnesses.	H	The government has reduced its expenditure in this area.
9	. . . Premature babies are **vulnerable** to illnesses.	I	But there are drugs which can slow down its cell-destroying properties.
10	. . . The National Health Service is suffering from **cutbacks** and **underfunding**.	J	Once the body's **cells** start growing abnormally, a cure can be difficult to find.
11	. . . The AIDS **virus** is **incurable**.	K	The pressures of a high-powered job can cause nervous **strain** which may require drugs.

Task 2: Replace the words or expressions in **bold** with a word or expression from the box which has the same meaning.

Cures

> • protein   • holistic medicine   • a diet   • minerals   • vitamins
> • therapeutic   • traditional medicines   • welfare state   • surgeon
> • active   • consultant   • conventional medicine

1 If you suffer from a bad back, a massage may be **able to cure or relieve the disorder**.

2 One of the secrets to remaining in good health is to choose **food to eat** that is high in fibre and low in fat.

3 Most people, when they are ill, rely on **modern pills and tablets** to cure them.

4 Some **old-fashioned cures for illnesses**, such as herbal tablets and remedies, are becoming increasingly popular.

5 Many people are turning to **treatments which involve the whole person, including their mental health, rather than just dealing with the symptoms of the illness**.

6 Doctors sometimes refer their patients to a **medical specialist attached to a hospital**.

7 It takes many years of training to become a **doctor specialising in surgery**.

8 Meat, eggs and nuts are rich sources of **a compound which is an essential part of living cells, and which is essential to keep the human body working properly**.

9 On his holiday, he had to take **essential substances which are not synthesised by the body but are found in food and are needed for growth and health**, because the food he ate lacked the B and C groups.

10 Calcium and zinc are two of the most important **substances found in food**.

11 Most doctors recommend an **energetic** lifestyle, with plenty of exercise.

12 British people enjoy free healthcare thanks to the **large amount of money which is spent to make sure they have adequate health services**.

Task 3: Now look at this extract from a magazine article and complete the gaps with one of the words or expressions from Tasks 1 and 2. In some cases, more than one answer may be possible. You may need to change the form of some of the words.

A cure for the future in the past?

For over fifty years, the people of Britain have relied on the (1) . . . . to make sure they have adequate health services. But now the National Health Service is sick. Government (2) . . . . and (3) . . . . are forcing hospitals to close, and waiting lists for treatment are getting longer. Under such circumstances, it is no surprise that more people are turning to private (but expensive) healthcare.

   For some, however, there are alternatives. They are turning their back on modern pills, tablets and other (4) . . . . It seems paradoxical, but in an age of microchips and high technology, (5) . . . . (the old-fashioned cures that our grandparents relied on) is making a comeback. Consider these case studies:

Healthcare

- Maude is 76 and has been suffering from (6) . . . . for almost ten years. 'The inflammation in my joints was almost unbearable, and my doctor referred me to a (7) . . . . at the London Hospital. I was told that I needed (8) . . . . , but would need to wait for at least two years before I could have the operation. In desperation, I started having massage sessions. To my surprise, these were very (9) . . . . , and while they didn't cure the disorder, they did relieve it to some extent.'

- Ron is 46. His high-powered city job was responsible for a series of (10) . . . . illnesses, and the drugs he took did little to relieve the nervous strain. 'I read about treatments which involve the whole person rather than the individual symptoms, but I had always been sceptical about (11) . . . . However, my friend recommended a dietician who advised me that part of my problem was (12) . . . . -related. Basically, the foods I was eating were contributing to my disorder. She gave me a list of foods that would provide the right (13) . . . . and (14) . . . . to keep me in good health. At the same time, she recommended a more (15) . . . . lifestyle – running, swimming, that kind of thing. I'm a bit of a couch potato, and the (16) . . . . lifestyle I had lived was compounding the problem. Now I feel great!'

So is there still a place in our lives for modern medicine? While it is true that some infections and viruses may be prevented by resorting to alternative medicine, more serious illnesses such as (17) . . . . need more drastic measures. We do need our health service at these times, and we shouldn't stop investing in its future. But we mustn't forget that for some common illnesses, the cure may lie in the past.

41 Travel

Task 1: Look at the following sentences and decide if they are **true** or **false**. If they are false, explain why.

1 A **travel agency** is the same as a **tour operator**.
2 A **package tour** is a holiday in which the price includes flights, transfers to and from the airport and accommodation.
3 An **all-inclusive** holiday is a holiday in which the price includes flights, transfers, accommodation, food and drink.
4 When passengers **embark**, they get *off* an aeroplane or ship.
5 When passengers **disembark**, they get *on* an aeroplane or ship.
6 The first thing you do when you go to an airport is go to the **check-in**.
7 The first thing you do when you arrive at your hotel is **check in**.
8 The opposite of a **package tourist** is an **independent traveller**.
9 **Mass tourism** can have a negative effect on the environment.
10 **Eco-tourism** is tourism which has a negative effect on the environment.
11 The words **trip**, **excursion**, **journey** and **voyage** all have the same meaning.
12 It is always necessary to have a **visa** when you visit a different country.
13 A flight from London to Paris could be described as a **long-haul** flight.
14 Flying **economy class** is more expensive than flying **business class**.
15 A Canadian citizen flying to Japan will have to fill in an **immigration card** before he arrives.

Task 2: Complete sentences 1–11 with a suitable word or expression from the box.

• **deported**	• **expatriates**	• **internally displaced**	• **repatriated**
• **immigration**	• **UNHCR**	• **persona non grata**	• **economic migrants**
• **culture shock**	• **emigration**	• **refugees**	

1 At the beginning of the war, thousands of . . . . fled over the border to the next country.
2 Since the civil war began, almost a million people have been forced to move to another part of the country. These . . . . persons are now without food or shelter.
3 Nineteenth-century governments encouraged . . . . to the colonies.
4 The government is encouraging . . . . because of the shortage of workers in key industries.
5 Going from California to live with hill tribes in India was something of a . . . .
6 Thousands of British . . . . live in Singapore, where many of them have high-powered jobs.
7 The . . . . is under a lot of pressure owing to the huge number of displaced persons around the world.
8 He was . . . . from the country when his visa expired.
9 Because he had a criminal record, the government didn't want him to enter the country, declared him . . . . and asked him to leave immediately.
10 After the economy collapsed in the east, thousands of . . . . headed west in the hope of finding a good job.
11 He didn't want to be . . . . , but nevertheless was put on a plane back home.

Task 3: Now look at this essay and complete the gaps with one of the words or expressions from Tasks 1 and 2. In some cases, more than one answer may be possible. You may need to change the form of some of the words.

Travel: the other side of the coin

Most of us have, at some point in our lives, experienced the joys of travel. We go to the (1) . . . . to pick up our brochures. We book a two-week (2) . . . . with flights and accommodation included (or if we are (3) . . . ., we make our own way to the country and travel around from place to place with a rucksack on our back). We make sure we have all the right currency, our passport and any (4) . . . . that are necessary to get us into the country. We go to the airport and (5) . . . . We strap ourselves into our tiny (6) . . . . aircraft seats and a few hours later we (7) . . . . from the aircraft, strange new sights, smells and sounds greeting us. Nowadays, it seems, the whole world goes on holiday at once: the age of (8) . . . . is in full swing!

But for the great majority of people around the world, travel for them is done in the face of great adversity and hardship. They never get to indulge in an (9) . . . . holiday in a luxury hotel with all meals and drinks included. They never get to explore the lush Amazon rain forest or the frozen wastes of the Arctic on an (10) . . . . holiday. For them, travel is a matter of life and death. I refer, of course, to all the (11) . . . . escaping from their own countries, or the (12) . . . ., moved from one part of their country to another by an uncaring government, or (13) . . . . forced to find a job and seek a living wherever they can.

Can you imagine anything worse than the misery these people must face? Let's not confuse them with those (14) . . . ., who choose to live in another country and often have nice houses and high salaries. These people are simply desperate to survive. As well as losing their homes because of war or famine or other natural disasters, they must come to terms with their new environment: for many, the (15) . . . . can be too great. And while many countries with an open policy on (16) . . . . will welcome them in with open arms, others will simply turn them away. These people become (17) . . . ., unwanted and unwelcome. Even if they manage to get into a country, they will often be (18) . . . . or repatriated. Their future is uncertain.

Something to think about, perhaps, the next time you are (19) . . . . to your five-star hotel by a palm-fringed beach or sitting in a coach on an (20) . . . . to a pretty castle in the countryside.

Don't forget to keep a record of the words and expressions that you have learnt, review your notes from time to time and try to use new vocabulary items whenever possible.

42 Crime and the law

Task 1: Match the words and expressions in the box with their correct definition 1–9.

> • **law-abiding**   • **solicitor**   • **defendant**   • **jury**   • **offender**   • **victim**
> • **barrister**   • **judge**   • **witness**

1 A person appointed to make legal decisions in a court of law.
2 A group of twelve citizens who are sworn to decide whether someone is guilty or innocent on the basis of evidence given in a court of law.
3 A person who sees something happen or is present when something happens.
4 A person who is accused of doing something illegal.
5 A person who is attacked or who is in an accident.
6 A qualified lawyer who gives advice to members of the public and acts for them in legal matters.
7 A person who commits an offence against the law.
8 A lawyer who can present a case in court.
9 An expression used to describe someone who obeys the law.

Task 2: The following groups of sentences describe the legal process which follows a crime. However, with the exception of the first sentence, the sentences in each group are in the wrong order. Put them into the correct order, using the key words in **bold** to help you. Some of these words appear in Task 1.

Part 1

A One night, Jim Smith committed a serious crime. (= Sentence 1)
B Jim asked the officer for a solicitor to help him.
C At the same time, the police arranged for a barrister to prosecute him.
D They took him to the police station and formally charged him with the crime.
E When the trial began and he appeared in court for the first time, he pleaded his innocence.
F The next morning the police arrested him.

Part 2

A His barrister also said he was **innocent** and asked the court to **acquit** him. (= Sentence 1)
B While he was in prison, he applied for **parole**.
C As a result, the judge **sentenced** him to two years in prison.
D He was **released** after 18 months.
E However, there were several **witnesses**, and the **evidence** against him was overwhelming.
F Having all the **proof** they needed, the **jury** returned a **guilty verdict**.

Part 3

A Unfortunately, prison failed to **rehabilitate** him and after his **release** he continued with his **misdeeds**, attacking an old woman in the street. (= Sentence 1)

B Jim promised to **reform** and the pensioner withdrew her call for more severe **retribution**.

C With this in mind, instead of passing a **custodial sentence**, he **fined** him a lot of money and ordered him to do **community service**.

D He was **re-arrested** and returned to court.

E His new **victim**, a pensioner, thought that the judge was being too **lenient** on Jim and called for the re-instatement of **corporal punishment** and **capital punishment**!

F At his second trial the judge agreed that prison was not a **deterrent** for Jim.

Task 3: Now look at this extract from a politician's speech and complete the gaps with one of the words or expressions from Tasks 1 and 2. In some cases, more than one answer may be possible. You may need to change the form of some of the words.

Are you worried about crime? I am. We read it every day in the papers. A terrible crime has been (1) . . . ., the police have (2) . . . . someone, he has appeared in front of a jury in (3) . . . ., he has (4) . . . . his innocence but has been found (5) . . . . of his crime and he has been (6) . . . . to ten years in prison. We are all very relieved that the criminal is being punished for his (7) . . . ., and (8) . . . . citizens like you and me can sleep more safely at night.

But what happens next? We all hope, don't we, that the prisoner will benefit from society's (9) . . . ., that a spell in prison will (10) . . . . him and make him a better person. We all hope that he will (11) . . . . and become like us. We all hope that when he is eventually (12) . . . . and let loose on the streets, he will be a good character, the threat of another spell in jail being a suitable (13) . . . . which will stop him from breaking the law again. Oh yes.

But let's face it. The reality is usually very different. The prisoner may be released on (14) . . . ., before the end of his sentence. He will try to re-enter society. But then he often becomes a (15) . . . . himself, unable to find work and rejected by society. It isn't long before he's back in prison again.

So what alternatives are there, I hear you say. What can we do to the (16) . . . . to make sure he doesn't commit another crime? There are alternatives to prison, of course, such as (17) . . . . in which he will provide a service to those around him. Or he can pay a large (18) . . . . Alternatively, we could establish a more severe system of punishment, including (19) . . . . and (20) . . . ., but we like to consider ourselves civilised, and the idea of beating or executing someone is repellent to us. Oh yes.

The answer, of course, is far simpler. We need to be tough not on the criminal, but on the cause of the crime. We should spend less of the taxpayer's money funding the (21) . . . . and (22) . . . . and all the other people who work for the legal system, and put the money instead into supporting deprived areas which are the breeding grounds for crime. We in the ConLab Party believe that everybody needs a good chance in life, and this is a good step forward. Vote for us now!

Don't forget to keep a record of the words and expressions that you have learnt, review your notes from time to time and try to use new vocabulary items whenever possible.

43 Social tensions

Task 1: Match each newspaper headline in the box with the first line of its accompanying story below. Use the words in **BOLD** to help you.

A **ILLEGAL ALIENS** TO BE EXPELLED
B **ETHNIC MINORITIES** 'LIVING BELOW **POVERTY** LEVEL'
C **HOMELESS SQUATTERS** EVICTED
D **INSTITUTIONAL RACISM** STILL A PROBLEM
E **INTERNALLY DISPLACED** IN NEW **GENOCIDE** HORROR
F **EXTREMISTS** ACCUSED OF PROMPTING **HOSTILITY**
G **UNREST**, **RIOTS** AND **ANARCHY** CONTINUE
H **REBELS** VICTORIOUS IN LATEST **POWER STRUGGLE**
I **DISCRIMINATION** AND **EXPLOITATION** A MAJOR PROBLEM IN BRITISH INDUSTRY
J **DISSIDENTS** ASK AUSTRALIAN GOVERNMENT FOR **POLITICAL ASYLUM**

1 Officers from the Thames Valley Police Force swooped on a house in Kidlington earlier this morning and forcibly removed a family who had been staying there illegally since they lost their home in August.

2 Almost 50% of factory workers in national companies claim they have received bad treatment or have been taken advantage of because of their class, religion, race , language, colour or sex, it has been revealed.

3 The UN has accused the government of Zarislavia of further atrocities committed in the west of the country, where hundreds of migrants are reported to have been killed by security forces.

4 Opponents of the government in Yugaria have asked to stay in Sydney because the political situation in their own country is making it unsafe for them to return.

5 The police have once again been accused of discriminating against minority groups, despite their reassurances earlier this year that they had reformed their practices.

6 Neo-Nazi groups in Paris were today condemned for inciting violence against non-whites in the centre of the city.

7 A shocking survey has revealed that almost 30% of Asian and African racial groups living in London are suffering financial hardship.

8 Following further devaluation of the Malovian dollar, violence has once again erupted on the streets of the capital.

9 Groups fighting against the government of George Malikes in Livatia have succeeded in capturing and occupying the parliament building.

10 The Government has ordered the immediate deportation of over 200 immigrants who entered the country without passports or visas last year.

Task 2: Match the words and expressions in the first box with a word or expression in the second box which is either the closest in meaning or which is normally associated with it. Some of these also appear in Task 1.

> • **ethnic cleansing**   • **prejudice**   • **civil rights**   • **harassment**   • **rebel**
> • **picket line**   • **poverty-stricken**   • **refugee**   • **outcast**

> • **reject** (noun)   • **non-conformist**   • **blackleg**   • **human rights**   • **destitute**
> • **discrimination**   • **displaced person**   • **intimidation**   • **racial purging**

Task 3: Now look at this news programme and complete the gaps with one of the words or expressions from Tasks 1 and 2. In some cases, more than one answer may be possible. You may need to change the form of some of the words.

Good evening. Here is the news.

Neo-Nazis and other (1) . . . . have been held responsible for a wave of (2) . . . . in the Bratilovan Republic. The United Nations estimates that over 20,000 people have been murdered there in the last six months. (3) . . . . who have escaped from the country have asked the British government to grant them (4) . . . ., as they fear for their safety if they have to return.

The government are to deport 500 (5) . . . . whose visas have expired. Angry members of the opposition have accused the government of (6) . . . ., as most of the deportees are of African origin. Meanwhile, the police have been accused of (7) . . . ., after Asian families in Bradford complained they had been pestered and worried by officers following a series of robberies in the city.

(8) . . . . leaders in the USA have held a demonstration in Washington against the death penalty. They have called for a total abolition of capital punishment, claiming that it is contrary to basic (9) . . . . principles outlined in the United Nations Declaration of Human Rights.

(10) . . . . fighting the government of President Stanislow have taken control of the television station in the centre of the capital. This follows a long-standing (11) . . . . between Mr Stanislow and the principal opposition party which has seriously weakened his power.

A spokesman for the (12) . . . . community in London has presented a petition to the government asking them to provide housing for everyone. He argues that the government's refusal to raise the minimum wage rate has resulted in thousands living in (13) . . . ., with not enough money to pay for somewhere to live. Meanwhile, the Metropolitan Police evicted several (14) . . . . who took over a house in the city centre last week and refused to leave until the government took positive action.

A recent survey reveals that at least 30% of public companies have been accused of (15) . . . . and (16) . . . . in the past year. The main offender is Anglo-Amalgamated Telecommunications, a Bristol-based company. Their employees, many of them Asian women, claim they have received bad treatment or been taken advantage of by the company.

And finally, the Cardiff police are preparing for angry scenes at the Welsh International Computers factory tomorrow when (17) . . . ., anxious to return to work after six months on strike, will attempt to break through the picket line. A senior officer has expressed his concern that there will be (18) . . . . and people will get hurt as a result.

44 Science and technology

Task 1: Replace the words and expressions in **bold** in sentences 1–18 with a word or expression from the box.

- analysed
- genetic engineering
- breakthrough
- molecular biology
- a technophobe
- safeguards
- development
- cybernetics
- invented
- nuclear engineering
- combined
- life expectancy
- discovered
- a technophile
- innovations
- react
- an experiment
- research

1 The company is carrying out **scientific study** to find a cure for AIDS.
2 The **planning and production** of the new computer system will take some time.
3 Modern home entertainment systems and other **modern inventions** are changing everyone's lives.
4 Some elements **change their chemical composition when mixed** with water.
5 The scientists have **created** a new machine to automate the process.
6 Who was the person who **found** penicillin.
7 When the food was **examined closely and scientifically**, it was found to contain bacteria.
8 Rain **joined together** with CO_2 gases produces acid rain.
9 Ron is **terrified of modern technology**.
10 Geoff is **very interested in modern technology**.
11 **Protection** against accidents in this laboratory are minimal.
12 Scientists conducted **a scientific test** to see how people react to different smells.
13 Brian is studying **the techniques used to change the genetic composition of a cell so as to change certain characteristics which can be inherited**.
14 Sarah is studying **the things which form the structure of living matter**.
15 Christine is studying **how information is communicated in machines and electronic devices in comparison with how it is communicated in the brain and nervous system**.
16 Neil is studying **the different ways of extracting and controlling energy from atomic particles**.
17 There has been a **sudden success** in the search for a cure for cancer.
18 **The number of years a person is likely to live** has increased a great deal thanks to modern medicine and technology.

Task 2: Read this description of a computer. Unfortunately, the person who is describing it is not very familiar with their computer vocabulary and cannot remember all the words. Help them by using the appropriate word or expression in the box to give a more scientific definition of their explanation.

• log on	• keyboard	• load	• e-mail	• download	• hardware
• crashed	• software	• the Internet	• scanner	• mouse	
• base unit/disk drive	• web site	• printer	• monitor		

OK, here's my new computer. As you can see, there are five main parts. Now this large box with the slots and sliding disc carrier is the most important part (1). It carries all the, eh, stuff that makes the computer work (2). You can also put in (3) your own games and other things (4). Next to it there is the thing that looks like a small television (5) so that you can see what the computer is doing. To the right of that, there is the machine that lets you make black and white or colour copies of the documents that you create on the computer (6). You can control the computer by using that rectangular flat thing with all the letters and numbers on (7) or that funny little object with the long lead which you can move across your desk (8). The large flat thing to the left of the computer is something you can use to make copies of your photographs or other documents onto the computer, a bit like a photocopier (9).

It's a very useful machine, of course. Once you, eh, get it up and running (10), you can do lots of things on it. You can create documents, play games or get information from this fantastic thing that links computers from around the world (11). A lot of companies and organisations have their own special computer page (12) which you can look at, and you can transfer the information (13) to your own computer files. Or, if you like, you can send messages to other people with computers by using this special facility called, eh, um, something I can't remember (14).

Unfortunately, I can't let you use it as it stopped working (15) last night. I think I must have done something wrong, but I can't imagine what. I've got a typewriter you can borrow if you like.

Task 3: Now look at this essay and fill in the gaps with one of the words or expressions from Tasks 1 and 2. In some cases, more than one answer may be possible. You may need to change some of the word forms.

Technology has come a long way in the last fifty years, and our lives have become better as a result. Or have they?

The second half of the twentieth century saw more changes than in the previous two hundred years. Penicillin has already been (1) . . . . and used to treat infections; there have been many remarkable advances in medicine that have helped to increase our average (2) . . . . way beyond that of our ancestors. Incredible (3) . . . . such as television have changed the way we spend our leisure hours. Perhaps the most important (4) . . . ., however, has been the microchip. Nobody could have imagined, when it was first (5) . . . ., that within a matter of years, this tiny piece of silicon and circuitry would be found in almost every household object from the kettle to the video recorder. And nobody could have predicted the sudden proliferation of computers that would completely change our lives, allowing us to access information from the other side of the world via the (6) . . . . or send messages around the world by (7) . . . . at the touch of a button. Meanwhile, (8) . . . . into other aspects of information technology is making it easier and cheaper for us to talk to friends and relations around the world. Good news for (9) . . . . who love modern technology, bad news for the (10) . . . . who would prefer to hide from these modern miracles.

But everything has a price. The development of (11) . . . . led to mass automation in factories, which in turn led to millions losing their jobs. The genius of Einstein led to the horrors of the atomic bomb and the dangerous uncertainties of (12) . . . . (we hear of accidents and mishaps at nuclear power stations around the world, where (13) . . . . to prevent accidents were inadequate). The relatively new science of (14) . . . . has been seen as a major step forward, but putting modified foods onto the market before scientists had properly (15) . . . . them was perhaps one of the most irresponsible decisions of the 1990s. Meanwhile, pharmaceutical companies continue to (16) . . . . on animals, a move that many consider to be cruel and unnecessary.

Of course we all rely on modern science and technology to improve our lives. However, we need to make sure that we can control it before it controls us.

Don't forget to keep a record of the words and expressions that you have learnt, review your notes from time to time and try to use new vocabulary items whenever possible.

45 Food and diet

Task 1: Find words in the word search grid below which have the same meaning as the dictionary definitions 1–11. A sample sentence with the word removed has been given to you.

1 Units of measurement of energy in food. (Example: **She's counting . . . . to try to lose weight.**)

2 A compound which is an essential part of living cells, one of the elements in food which you need to keep the human body working properly. (Example: **Eggs are a rich source of . . . .**)

3 A chemical substance containing carbon, hydrogen and oxygen. (Example: **Bread, potatoes and rice are good sources of . . . .**)

4 A white substance from plants or animals which can be used for cooking. (Example: **Fry the meat and drain off the . . . .**)

5 Matter in food which cannot be digested and passes out of the body. (Example: **A diet that doesn't contain enough . . . . can cause intestinal problems.**)

6 A fatty substance found in fats and oils, also produced by the liver and forming an essential part of all cells. (Example: **If you eat too much . . . . , it can be deposited on the walls of arteries, causing them to become blocked.**)

7 Essential substance which is not synthesised by the body but is found in food and is needed for health and growth. (Example: **He doesn't eat enough fruit and suffers from . . . . C deficiency.**)

8 Substance which is found in food, but which can also be dug out of the earth. (Example: **What is the . . . . content of spinach?**)

9 Too heavy, often as a result of eating too much. (Example: **The doctor says I'm . . . . and must go on a diet.**)

10 The result of not having enough to eat, or the result of eating too much of the wrong sort of food. (Example: **Many of the children in the refugee camp were . . . .**)

11 Receiving food. (Example: **We are developing a scheme to improve . . . . in the poorer areas.**)

W	E	C	R	T	Y	U	H	F	V	F	H	E	N
M	C	A	R	B	O	H	Y	D	R	A	T	E	S
Y	S	L	C	E	A	C	Z	Q	W	T	E	R	T
U	I	O	H	E	R	V	Z	X	C	V	B	N	M
A	P	R	O	T	E	I	N	A	D	F	G	H	J
K	L	I	L	N	U	T	R	I	T	I	O	N	M
C	V	E	E	B	N	A	Z	X	C	V	B	N	M
L	K	S	S	J	H	M	I	N	E	R	A	L	B
M	N	B	T	V	C	I	L	K	J	H	G	F	D
U	Y	T	E	W	E	N	R	T	Y	U	I	O	P
F	I	B	R	E	A	E	Q	W	E	D	G	T	X
H	E	D	O	V	E	R	W	E	I	G	H	T	B
C	M	A	L	N	O	U	R	I	S	H	E	D	Y
Q	W	E	G	S	T	C	V	T	W	R	D	W	T

Task 2: Match sentences 1–10 with a second sentence A–J. Use the key words in **bold** to help you.

1 A lot of people are **allergic** to nuts.
2 Many people do not trust **genetically modified** foods.
3 **Organic** vegetables are more expensive but are better for you.
4 We refuse to eat **battery chickens**.
5 We prefer to eat **free range** meats.
6 The **harvest** has been very bad this year.
7 Following the floods in Mozambique, there was a terrible **scarcity** of food.
8 There has been an outbreak of **salmonella**, **listeria** and other **food poisoning** in Perth.
9 Too many people don't eat a **balanced diet**.
10 **Fast food** is very popular.

A This is because they are cultivated naturally, without using any chemical fertilisers and pesticides.
B There wasn't enough to feed everyone affected by the disaster.
C They are not sure that altering the composition of cells to change certain characteristics is safe.
D It's good to know that the animals were given enough space to express their natural behaviour.
E Terrible weather conditions have prevented the crops from ripening and reduced the yield.
F A lot of people are in hospital as a result.
G Unfortunately, a diet of burgers, pizzas and fried chicken is not very healthy.
H They physically react very badly.
I This is because they spend their life confined in a small cage.
J They don't consume sufficient quantities of the different food groups.

Task 3: Now complete this article with one of the words or expressions from Tasks 1 and 2. In some cases, more than one answer may be possible. You may need to change some of the word forms.

Most children enjoy eating (1) . . . . , but scientific tests have shown us that burgers and pizzas can lack essential (2) . . . . and (3) . . . . which are essential for health and growth, while simultaneously containing large amounts of (4) . . . . and (5) . . . . which can result in obesity and heart problems. Many children end up suffering from (6) . . . . , since they eat too much of the wrong sort of food. In fact, in many areas of the developed world, a lot of children show similar symptoms to those in poorer developing countries, where (7) . . . . of food causes thousands of deaths from starvation, especially in the wake of natural disasters which ruin crops and in some cases totally destroy the annual (8) . . . .

Dieticians tell us that we must eat a (9) . . . . , as it is essential we consume sufficient quantities of the different food groups. They tell us that we should all eat more (10) . . . . , which cannot be digested by the body, and fewer foods which are high in (11) . . . . , as this can block the walls of arteries and lead to heart problems. This is good advice, of course, but our lifestyles often make this difficult. Many of the ready-prepared foods we buy from supermarkets are high in (12) . . . ., giving us more energy than we actually need. (13) . . . . foods are appearing on our supermarket shelves, even though nobody is really sure if altering the composition of food cells is safe. We have the option, of course, of buying (14) . . . . foods, but naturally-cultivated fruits and vegetables are expensive. And to make matters worse, we are continually hearing about outbreaks of (15) . . . . and (16) . . . . which put us off eating certain foods, as nobody wants to spend time in hospital suffering from (17) . . . .

A few things to watch out for next time you go shopping. If you have the time and the money, that is!

46 Children and the family

Task 1: Complete these sentences with an appropriate word or expression from A, B or C.

1 Mr and Mrs Smith live at home with their two children. They are a typical example of a modern . . . . family.
   A. extended   **B. nuclear**   **C. compact**

2 Mr and Mrs Popatlal live at home with their aged parents, children and grandchildren. They are a typical example of a traditional . . . . family.
   A. nuclear   **B. enlarged**   **C. extended**

3 Mrs Jones lives on her own and has to look after her two children. There are a lot of . . . . families like hers.
   A. single-parent   **B. mother-only**   **C. mono-parent**

4 Some parents need to . . . . their children more strictly.
   A. bring down   **B. bring about**   **C. bring up**

5 When I was a child, I had a very turbulent . . . .
   A. upbringing   **B. upraising**   **C. uplifting**

6 Mrs Kelly is . . . . and finds it difficult to look after her children on her own.
   A. divorced   **B. divided**   **C. diverged**

7 Many men believe that . . . . is the responsibility of a woman.
   A. childhelp   **B. childcare**   **C. childaid**

8 . . . . is a particularly difficult time of life for a child.
   A. convalescence   **B. adolescence**   **C. convergence**

9 A person's behaviour can sometimes be traced back to his/her . . . .
   A. creative years   **B. formulating years**   **C. formative years**

10 The country has seen a sharp drop in the . . . . in the last few years.
   A. birth rate   **B. baby rate**   **C. born rate**

11 She has five . . . . who rely on her to look after them.
   A. dependants   **B. dependers**   **C. dependents**

12 . . . . is on the rise, with over 20% of serious crimes being committed by children under the age of seventeen.
   A. junior crime   **B. juvenile delinquency**   **C. minor crime**

Task 2: Match sentences 1–12 with a second sentence A–L. Use the key words in **bold** to help you.

1 Mr and Mrs White are very **authoritarian** parents.

2 Mr Bowles is considered to be too **lenient**.

3 Mr and Mrs Harris lead **separate lives**.

4 Billy is a **well-adjusted** kid.

5 The Mannings are not very **responsible** parents.

6 My parents are **separated**.

7 Parents must look after their children, but they shouldn't be **over-protective**.

8 Professor Maynard has made a study of the **cognitive processes** of young children.

9 I'm afraid my youngest child is **running wild**.

10 She looks quite different from all her **siblings**.

11 There are several different and distinct **stages of development** in a child's life.

12 Tony was raised by a **foster family** when his own parents died.

A They don't look after their children very well.

B He is fascinated by the way they learn new things.

C He very rarely punishes his children.

D I live with my mother and visit my father at weekends.

E He never listens to a word I say, and is always playing truant from school.

F Brothers and sisters usually bear some resemblance to one another.

G Although they are married and live together, they rarely speak to each other.

H They are very strict with their children.

I Of all of these, the teenage years are the most difficult.

J Children need the freedom to get out and experience the world around them.

K He's happy at home and is doing well at school.

L My families take in children who are not their own.

Task 3: Now read this case study and fill in the gaps with one of the words or expressions from Tasks 1 and 2. In some cases, more than one answer may be possible. You may need to change some of the word forms.

Bob's problems began during his (1) . . . . years. His parents got (2) . . . . when he was young, and neither of his parents wanted to raise him or his brother and sister, so he was (3) . . . . by a (4) . . . . chosen by his parent's social worker. Unfortunately, his foster-father was a strict (5) . . . . and often beat him. Bob rebelled against this strict (6) . . . . , and by the time he was eight, he was already (7) . . . . , stealing from shops and playing truant. By the time he reached (8) . . . . , sometime around his thirteenth birthday, he had already appeared in court several times, charged with (9) . . . . The judge blamed his foster-parents, explaining that children needed (10) . . . . parents and guardians who would look after them properly. The foster-father objected to this, pointing out that Bob's (11) . . . . – his two brothers and sister – were (12) . . . . children who behaved at home and worked well at school.

  This has raised some interesting questions about the modern family system. While it is true that parents should not be too (13) . . . . with children by letting them do what they want when they want, or be too (14) . . . . by sheltering them from the realities of life, it is also true that they should not be too strict. It has also highlighted the disadvantages of the modern (15) . . . . family where the child has only its mother and father to rely on (or the (16) . . . . family, in which the mother or father has to struggle particularly hard to support their (17) . . . .). In fact, many believe that we should return to traditional family values and the (18) . . . . family: extensive research has shown that children from these families are generally better behaved and have a better chance of success in later life.

47 On the road

Task 1: Choose the most suitable explanation, A or B, for the following sentences. Use the words in **bold** to help you.

1 People enjoy the **mobility** that owning a car gives them.
   A. *People enjoy being able to travel easily from one place to another.*
   B. *People enjoy being able to drive very fast.*

2 What's your **destination**?
   A. *Where have you come from?*
   B. *Where are you going to?*

3 **Congestion** in the city centre has increased dramatically.
   A. *It is now easier to drive around the city centre than it was before.*
   B. *It is now more difficult to drive around the city centre than it was before.*

4 The local council wants to reduce the risks to **pedestrians**.
   A. *The local council wants to make it safer for people to walk along the street.*
   B. *The local council wants to make it safer for drivers and their passengers.*

5 Lead-free petrol reduces the risk of **pollution**.
   A. *Lead-free petrol does not make the environment as dirty as conventional petrol.*
   B. *Cars fuelled by lead-free pollution are safer to drive.*

6 **Traffic-calming** measures are becoming increasingly common throughout the country.
   A. *People have to drive more slowly because of the increased number of police in villages and towns.*
   B. *People have to drive more carefully through towns and villages because of specially-built obstacles in the road.*

7 The centre of Camford has been designated a **traffic-free zone**.
   A. *You cannot take your car into the centre of Camford.*
   B. *You can park your car for free in the centre of Camford.*

8 Container lorries and other large vehicles **dominate** our roads.
   A. *There are a lot of large vehicles on the roads.*
   B. *There aren't many large vehicles on the roads.*

9 Young drivers have a higher **accident risk** than older drivers.
   A. *Young drivers are more likely than older drivers to be involved in a crash.*
   B. *Young drivers are less likely than older drivers to be involved in a crash.*

10 Public transport is heavily **subsidised** in most areas.
   A. *The government has made public transport cheaper to use by giving money to bus and train companies.*
   B. *The government has made public transport more expensive to use by increasing the price of road tax.*

11 The junction of London Road and Holly Street is an accident **black spot**.
   A. *A lot of traffic accidents happen here.*
   B. *Not many accidents happen here.*

12 The city council needs to adopt an effective **transport strategy** within the next five years.
   A. *The city council needs to find a better way for people to get into, around and out of the city.*
   B. *The city council needs to encourage more drivers to bring their cars into the city.*

Task 2: Look at sentences 1–10 and decide what has, or hasn't, happened (sentences A–J). Use the words in **bold** to help you.

1 *Ambulance driver to policeman:* 'The pedestrian's **injuries** are very severe and he has to go to hospital.'
2 *Judge to driver:* '**Drink-driving** is a serious offence and I therefore ban you from driving for a year.'
3 *Driving instructor to student driver:* 'Stop! That's a **pedestrian crossing**!'
4 *Driving test examiner to student driver:* 'I'm afraid you've failed your test because you don't know the **Highway Code**.'
5 *Policeman to driver:* 'Do you realise you were **speeding** back there, sir?'
6 *Driver to a friend:* 'I can't believe it! He gave me a heavy **fine** and six points on my licence.'
7 *Police officer to radio interviewer:* '**Joyriding** has increased by almost 50% and I am urging everyone to think twice before they get involved in this stupid activity.'
8 *Television news presenter:* 'So far this year there have been 27 **fatalities** on Oxfordshire's roads.'
9 *City council officer to journalist:* 'As part of our new transport strategy, we are going to construct **cycle lanes** in and around the city.'
10 *City council officer to journalist:* 'The "**Park and Ride**" scheme has been very successful over the last year.'

A Somebody is unfamiliar with the government publication containing the rules for people travelling on roads.
B More people have been leaving their cars in designated areas outside a city and catching a bus into the city centre.
C A lot of cars have been stolen, mainly by young people who want some excitement.
D A person walking in the street has been hit and badly hurt by a vehicle.
E Somebody has decided to make it safer to use bicycles.
F Somebody has almost driven through a red light and hit a person walking across the road.
G Somebody has had to pay money because of a driving offence.
H Somebody has consumed an illegal amount of alcohol before driving their car.
I A lot of people have been killed in traffic-related accidents.
J Somebody has been driving too fast.

Task 3: Now read this article and fill in the gaps with one of the words or expressions from Tasks 1 and 2. In some cases, more than one answer may be possible. You may need to change some of the word forms.

(1) . . . . and (2) . . . . on Britain's roads are increasing from year to year: last year, 2,827 people were killed and almost 300,000 hurt in traffic-related accidents. Most of these were caused by drivers (3) . . . . in built-up areas, where many seem to disregard the 30 mph limit, or (4) . . . ., especially around Christmas, when more alcohol is consumed than at any other time. In many cases, it is (5) . . . . who are the victims, knocked down as they are walking across the street at (6) . . . . by drivers who seem to have forgotten that the rules of the (7) . . . . order you to stop at red lights.

But these innocent victims, together with the help of the police and local councils, are fighting back. In Oxford, a city plagued by (8) . . . . and (9) . . . . caused by traffic, and a notorious accident (10) . . . . for pedestrians and cyclists, the city council has recently implemented its new (11) . . . . , which has improved the flow of traffic to the benefit of those on foot or on two wheels. (12) . . . . measures such as bollards and speed humps have slowed traffic down. (13) . . . . schemes have helped reduce the number of cars in the city, as office workers and shoppers leave their cars outside the city and bus in instead. Cornmarket Street, the main shopping thoroughfare, has been designated a (14) . . . . , closed to all vehicles during the day. There are more (15) . . . . on main routes into the city, making it safer for the huge number of students and residents who rely on bicycles to get around. And (16) . . . . public transport has helped to keep down the cost of using buses. Meanwhile, the police and the courts are coming down hard on drivers who misuse the roads, handing down large (17) . . . . on selfish, inconsiderate drivers who believe it is their right to (18) . . . . the roads.

Task 1: Look at sentences 1–10, which are all extracts from art reviews, and decide what is being talked about in each one. Choose the most appropriate answer from the box. There are some which are not needed.

Performing arts
- a modern dance piece
- a concert
- a play
- an opera
- a film
- a ballet

Literature
- poetry
- a biography
- drama
- a novel
- a collection of short stories

Fine/visual arts
- abstract art
- a landscape
- a portrait
- a still life
- a sculpture

1 Mimi Latouche is getting a little too old for this kind of thing, and as I watched her pirouette across the stage in a tutu two sizes too small, she reminded me not so much of a swan as a rather ungainly crow.

2 The scenery was wonderful. The costumes were marvellous. The cast were incredible. I wish I could say the same about the script. The playwright should be shot.

3 In his new book on Ernest Hemingway, acclaimed writer Michael Norris has brought the great man to life in a way nobody else could.

4 Move over Michelangelo! You have a rival. Vittorio Manelleto's marble pieces embody the human form in a way that has not been achieved in over five hundred years.

5 I had to study the picture for almost two minutes before I realised who it was. It was none other than our Queen. I doubt she would have been amused.

6 There are no great tenors in Britain. That is until now. Brian Clack's performance in La Traviata sent shudders down my spine. What a man! What a voice! What a size!

7 Herbert von Caravan has been conducting now for almost forty years, and his final appearance yesterday was greeted with remarkable applause from both musicians and members of the audience.

8 'Stone Angel' is an hilarious tale about the fall and rise of an opera singer. I picked it up and didn't put it down until I had finished. A fantastic book.

9 Dylan Thomas showed remarkable eloquence, and this latest compilation of some of his finest verse will surely be a bestseller.

10 Bruschetta's studies of dead animals might not be to everyone's taste, but it is impossible to deny his skill in representing inanimate objects like these on canvas.

Task 2: Complete these sentences with an appropriate word or expression from A, B or C.

1 Tonight's . . . . of 'Hamlet' begins at 7.30.
   A. perform   **B. performing**   **C. performance**

2 Camford University Press have just released a collection of Shakespeare's . . . .
   A. works   **B. workers**   **C. workings**

3 The rock group 'Glass Weasel' have released a limited . . . . of their new album which contains a CD-ROM of their latest show.
   A. edit   **B. edition**   **C. editor**

4 His last book received excellent . . . . in the newspapers.
   A. reviews   **B. previews**   **C. revisions**

5 There is an . . . . of Monet's work at the Tate.
   A. exhibitionist   **B. exhibit**   **C. exhibition**

6 The British National Orchestra is delighted with the government's promise of a £500,000 . . . .
   A. subsidiary   **B. subsidy**   **C. subpoena**

7 Tickets have already sold out for the first day's showing of Tom Cartmill's paintings at the National . . . .
   A. Galleon   **B. Galley**   **C. Gallery**

8 Ernest Hemingway was one of the twentieth century's most famous . . . .
   A. novels   **B. novelties**   **C. novelists**

9 The French . . . . of the nineteenth century had a profound influence on the world of art.
   A. impressions   **B. impressionists**   **C. impressionisms**

10 Oldhaven Press are going to . . . . my new book!
   A. publish   **B. publisher**   **C. publication**

Task 3: Now look at this extract from a radio programme and fill in the gaps with one of the words or expressions from Tasks 1 and 2. In some cases, more than one answer may be possible. You may need to change some of the word forms.

Hello, and welcome to today's edition of 'But is it Art?'

Now, I don't usually enjoy (1) . . . . – all those pirouettes and *pas de deuxs* and dying swans usually send me to sleep, but last night's (2) . . . . of 'Sleeping Beauty' at Nureyev Hall had me on the edge of my seat. And I'm not the only one: rave (3) . . . . in the national press praised the excellent choreography and the incredible stage set. It's on again tonight, but you'll have to move fast if you want a ticket!

The current (4) . . . . of Monetto's paintings at the Wheatley (5) . . . . has been a disappointment. The pictures themselves are excellent, especially the great artist's (6) . . . . of film stars, and of course his stunning (7) . . . . of a vase of daffodils, but the lighting inside the room was terrible. I would have thought that, having received a government (8) . . . . of almost £100,000, the Wheatley Arts Council could have invested it in some good lights.

Fans of the great twentieth century (9) . . . . George Orwell will be delighted to hear that Swansong Press are going to release a collection of his greatest (10) . . . ., which will of course include *Animal Farm* and *Nineteen Eighty Four*. Also included are some rare short stories which were not (11) . . . . until after his death. Look out for the book, which will be in the shops from the end of the month.

On the subject of books, a new (12) . . . . of the life of conductor Charles Worsenmost is due to be released in January. Worsenmost conducted his last (13) . . . . in 1998 after a long and eventful career. This is highly recommended for anyone who is remotely interested in classical music.

Have you ever wanted to be an (14) . . . . singer? Well, now's your chance! The National Music Company are looking for tenors and sopranos to audition for a new production of Mozart's 'Marriage of Figaro'. If you're interested, we'll give you the number to call at the end of the programme.

Potential Michelangelos and Henry Moores can try their hand at (15) . . . . this weekend. The Gleneagles Museum is holding a series of workshops which will give you the chance to chip away at a lump of stone to produce a piece of three-dimensional art. There's no need to book – just turn up at the door on Saturday at nine o'clock.

And now here's that number I promised you . . .

Don't forget to keep a record of the words and expressions that you have learnt, review your notes from time to time and try to use new vocabulary items whenever possible.

Task 1: Match the sentences in the left-hand column with the most appropriate sentence in the right-hand column. Use the words in **bold** to help you.

1	London is a truly **cosmopolitan** city.	A	**Drug abuse** is also a big problem.
2	A modern **metropolis** needs a good integrated transport system.	B	Shops, libraries, hospitals and entertainment complexes are just a few of them.
3	London suffers a lot from traffic **congestion**.	C	Chief among these are concerts and exhibitions.
4	**Poverty** in the **inner-city** areas can **breed crime**.	D	In particular, I enjoy the **atmosphere** that is unique to the city.
5	Cities around the world have seen a huge **population explosion**.	E	Prices in London are particularly exorbitant.
6	Birmingham has plenty of **amenities**.	F	Without them, they are unable to function properly as cities.
7	A lot of people visit Paris for its **cultural events**.	G	It is especially bad during the **rush hour**, when thousands of **commuters** try to enter or leave the city.
8	Cities in poorer countries often lack basic **infrastructures**.	H	Stress-related illnesses are very common in cities like New York.
9	The **pressures of modern city life** can be difficult to deal with.	I	Nowadays there are more **city dwellers** than ever before.
10	The **cost of living** in some places can be very high.	J	Everywhere you go there are **building sites**, **pedestrian precincts**, **blocks of flats** and **housing estates** spreading into the countryside.
11	A lot of people appreciate the **anonymity** of living in a large city.	K	They like to feel that they can do something without everybody knowing about it.
12	I love the **urban lifestyle** I lead.	L	Most people use buses and the underground to get to the banks and offices where they work.
13	In Singapore, private cars are banned from the **Central Business District** at **peak periods**.	M	Unfortunately, this is something that most large capital cities lack.
14	**Urban sprawl** is prevalent in most cities.	N	It's a **melting pot** for people from all parts of the world.

Task 2: Match the sentences in the left-hand column with an appropriate response in the right-hand column. Use the words in **bold** to help you.

1	I enjoy a **rural** lifestyle.	A	Really? So why are we seeing so much **construction** in the countryside around London?
2	There isn't much **pollution** if you live outside a town.	B	I'm not so sure. All those **pesticides** and **chemical fertilisers** that farmers use nowadays can't be good for the **environment**.
3	There is a lot of **productive land** in this area.	C	That's probably because we import more food from abroad.
4	In recent years, there has been a lot of **migration** from the towns to the cities.	D	Mostly **wheat**, **oats** and **barley**.
5	The government has promised to leave the **green belt** alone.	E	Really? How much is that in **acres**?
6	There has been a huge reduction in the amount of **arable land** over the last twenty years.	F	I'm not surprised. With such terrible **prospects** within towns, **depopulation** is inevitable.
7	My uncle's farm covers almost 800 **hectares**.	G	Well I can't see much evidence of **cultivation**.
8	What are the main **crops** grown in this area?	H	Really? I always find there's nothing to do in the countryside.

Task 3: Now read this article and fill in the gaps with one of the words or expressions from Tasks 1 and 2. In some cases, more than one answer may be possible. You may need to change some of the word forms.

For seven years I lived in Singapore, a (1) . . . . of almost three million people. Like London, Paris and New York, Singapore is a (2) . . . . city, with people from different parts of the world living and working together. I enjoyed the (3) . . . . lifestyle I led there, and made the most of the superb (4) . . . ., ranging from the excellent shops to some of the best restaurants in the world. In the evenings and at weekends there were always (5) . . . .; with such diverse attractions as classical western music, an exhibition of Malay art or a Chinese opera in the street, it was difficult to get bored. Perhaps most impressive, however, was the remarkable transport (6) . . . ., with excellent roads, a swift and efficient bus service and a state-of-the-art underground system which could whisk (7) . . . . from the suburbs straight into the heart of the city (this was particularly important, as the government banned private cars from entering the (8) . . . . during the morning and afternoon (9) . . . . in order to reduce (10) . . . . on the roads and (11) . . . . from the exhausts.

Of course, living in a city like this has its disadvantages as well. For a start, the (12) . . . . can be very high – renting an apartment, for example, is very expensive. And as the city is expanding, there are a lot of (13) . . . . where new apartments are continually being built to deal with the (14) . . . . which is a direct result of the government encouraging people to have more children.

Fortunately, Singapore doesn't suffer from problems that are common in many cities such as (15) . . . . , which is partly the result of the government imposing very severe penalties on anyone bringing narcotics into the country, so it is safe to walk the streets at night. In fact, the (16) . . . . housing estates there are probably the safest and most orderly in the world.

Singapore wouldn't be ideal for everyone, however, especially if you come from the countryside and are used to a (17) . . . . lifestyle. The traditional villages that were once common have disappeared as the residents there realised there were no (18) . . . . for their future and moved into new government housing in the city. Nowadays, there is very little (19) . . . . around the city, which means that Singapore imports almost all of its food. And despite a 'green' approach to city planning, the (20) . . . . which has eaten into the countryside has had a detrimental effect on the (21) . . . .

Don't forget to keep a record of the words and expressions that you have learnt, review your notes from time to time and try to use new vocabulary items whenever possible.

50 Architecture

Task 1: Put the words in the box into their appropriate category in the table beneath. Some words can go into more than one category.

> - modernist   • reinforced concrete   • practical   • post-modern
> - standardised   • skyscraper   • well-designed   • porch   • façade
> - traditional   • walls   • an eyesore   • timber   • elegant   • stone
> - steel   • functional   • ugly   • glass   • concrete   • low-rise apartments
> - high-tech   • controversial   • high-rise apartments   • pleasing geometric forms
> - art deco   • multi-storey car park   • international style   • energy-efficient
> - foundations

Building materials (6 words/expressions)	Aesthetic perception (how we feel about a building) (6 words/expressions)
Types of building (4 words/expressions)	Architectural style (6 words/expressions)
Parts of a building (4 words/expressions)	Features (that make the building easy to live or work in) (4 words/expressions)

Task 2: (Level: Intermediate/Upper-intermediate): Complete these sentences with an appropriate word or expression from A, B or C.

1 The building is . . . . It's been ruined and abandoned for years.
   A. destabilised   **B. derelict**   **C. defunct**

2 She lives on a large housing . . . . near the centre of the city.
   A. estate   **B. state**   **C. estuary**

3 There are several dirty districts inside the city, although most of these . . . . are going to be replaced by high-rise apartments.
   A. slumps   **B. scrums**   **C. slums**

4 The city council are going to . . . . the old church and built a new one in its place.
   A. demobilise   **B. demote**   **C. demolish**

5 You can't knock down that house; there's a . . . . order on it which makes it illegal to destroy it.
   A. preservation   **B. preservative**   **C. presentable**

6 Sir Richard Rogers is the . . . . who designed the Lloyds building in London.
   A. architect   **B. architecture**   **C. architectural**

7 Some of the problems in our . . . . are drug-related.
   A. inter-cities   **B. internal cities**   **C. inner-cities**

8 The council hope to reduce crime in the town by introducing new . . . . facilities so that people have something to do in the evening.
   A. sociable   **B. socialist**   **C. social**

9 The cinema is going to be closed for two months while the owners . . . . it.
   A. renovate   **B. remonstrate**   **C. reiterate**

10 If you want to add an extension to your house, you will need . . . . permission from your local council.
   A. planning   **B. construction**   **C. plotting**

Task 3: Now look at this report and fill in the gaps with one of the words or expressions from Tasks 1 and 2. In some cases, more than one answer may be possible. You may need to change some of the word forms.

Report from the director of the West Twyford Town Planning Committee

The last year has been a busy one for the West Twyford Town Planning Committee. Outlined below are a few of the areas we have concentrated on.

1 Applications for (1) . . . . permission from home owners who want to develop their properties have increased by 50%. However, many of these homes are historic buildings and have (2) . . . . orders which prevent them from being altered externally. At present, we can only allow owners to (3) . . . . the inside of their homes (including installing central heating and improved wall insulation).

2 Last summer we invited several (4) . . . . to design plans for the new council offices on Peach Street. We eventually chose Barnard, Jackson and Willis, a local company. It was generally agreed that their design, which included a grey tinted (5) . . . . (6) . . . . at the front of the building, was the most aesthetically pleasing. They are currently in the process of laying the (7) . . . . for the new building, which we understand is taking some time as the land must be drained first.

3 In response to a lot of complaints about the lack of (8) . . . . facilities in the town, it was agreed at last month's meeting that funds should be set aside for the construction of a new sports centre and youth club.

4 Several (9) . . . . buildings which have been ruined and abandoned for over five years are to be knocked down. In their place, a new housing (10) . . . . will be built. This will provide twenty new homes within the next two years.

5 Everybody agrees that the new shops on the High Street are (11) . . . . It is certainly true that they are very ugly and out of keeping with the other buildings on the street. In future, we must ensure that all new buildings are built in a (12) . . . . style so that they fit in with the older buildings around them.

6 There has been an increased crime rate in the (13) . . . . to the east of the town. We plan to demolish these dirty areas within the next eight years and re-house the residents in new (14) . . . . apartments in the Berkely Heath district.

7 In an attempt to help the environment, we are going to make the town hall more (15) . . . . Windows will be double-glazed, walls and ceilings will be insulated and we will replace the current central heating system.

My next report will be in two months' time. Anybody wishing to discuss these issues can contact me on extension 287.

Don't forget to keep a record of the words and expressions that you have learnt, review your notes from time to time and try to use new vocabulary items whenever possible.

51 Men and women

Task 1: Look at the words and expressions in **bold** in the following sentences and decide if we generally consider them to have a <u>positive</u> connotation or a <u>negative</u> connotation.

1 At the interview, the manager was impressed by her **astute** comments.

2 In the **power struggle** between men and women, neither side will win.

3 After the takeover, the staff hoped that things would improve, but the new manager was just as **ruthless** as the man he replaced.

4 Some men believe that women are the **weaker sex** and should leave real work to men.

5 Our boss is a **male chauvinist** and believes that women should get less money than men for the same job.

6 John doesn't consider women to be very intelligent. To him, they are just **sex objects**.

7 Our company is **male-dominated**; all the top management positions are occupied by men.

8 Maureen is a **multi-faceted** worker. She is able to do a number of different jobs, often at the same time.

9 He holds **egalitarian** views and believes that everybody should be treated equally.

10 The new management has taken steps to ensure **equality** in the office; from now on, everyone will receive the same money regardless of their sex or age.

11 **Militant feminists** have thrown paint at a well-known television personality in order to stress their views.

	Positive	Negative
1		
2		
3		
4		
5		
6		
7		
8		
9		

Task 2: Use the words and expressions in the box to complete the conversation below.

> • gender roles   • child-rearing   • male counterparts   • breadwinner
> • stereotypes   • household management   • role division   • battle of the sexes
> • Sex Discrimination Act   • social convention

Chris: Cleaning and cooking are a woman's job. After all, men are no good at (1) . . . .

Terry: What rubbish! Thank goodness the (2) . . . . exists to prevent men from taking advantage of women.

Chris: Well, let's face it, in the workplace women never do as well as their (3) . . . .

Terry: And I suppose you think that women are only good for changing babies' nappies and other tedious aspects of (4) . . . .

Chris: No, but I do believe that in a modern household there should be a clearly-defined (5) . . . . Men are good at DIY, for example. Most women aren't. And I'll always believe that it's the man who should be the (6) . . . . , providing food and shelter for his family.

Terry: Well, all I can say is that I'm glad your ideas of (7) . . . . are not shared by most people.

Chris: Nonsense! A lot of people believe in traditional (8) . . . . ; the man goes out to work, the woman stays at home. It's as simple as that.

Terry: Men at work and women at home? Come on dear, those are such typical (9) . . . . ! With people like you around, the (10) . . . . will always continue.

Chris: Oh, shut up dad.

Terry: Sorry Christine, but it's an issue I feel strongly about.

Task 3: Now read this essay and complete the gaps with one of the words or expressions from Tasks 1 and 2.

'Men and women are, and always will be, different in the way they behave and are treated'. Do you agree with this statement?

A totally (1) . . . . society, in which sexual (2) . . . . between men and women is the norm, is still a long way off. This is certainly the case if you watch television, where men are often portrayed as the (3) . . . . , bringing money home to the wife, who is usually depicted as the (4) . . . . , prone to extreme emotions and temper tantrums. But is this really the case? Is it still fair to create (5) . . . . such as this? After all, as more women go out to work and more men stay at home to look after the house and the kids, it is quite clear that so-called (6) . . . . are merging and disappearing.

Take the office workplace as an example. For years, businesses and companies were (7) . . . . – the directors, managers and businessmen were always men, the secretaries and personal assistants always female. This was probably because men have traditionally been seen as more (8) . . . . , more able to deal with the cut-and-thrust of business. But now women are proving that they can be equally tough, while simultaneously being more (9) . . . . and caring. In fact, in many ways, women are more (10) . . . . than men, a vital aspect of modern

business where you are expected to do more than just one job. And thanks to the (11) . . . . ,
women are paid the same as men. It would appear that, in many cases, the (12) . . . . is a
dying breed.

At home, too, there is less evidence of (13) . . . . It is no longer the woman who does all
the cooking and cleaning and (14) . . . . Such (15) . . . . is now often shared
equally. (16) . . . . no longer requires the woman to stay indoors all day while the man stays
out until all hours. Whether this is due to the struggle by the (17) . . . . in the 1960s and
1970s, or whether it is due to a natural shift in attitudes is unclear.

What is clear, however, is that women no longer feel they need to be regarded as
(18) . . . . , the underdogs in a (19) . . . . with their (20) . . . . In fact,
many believe that in the (21) . . . . , it is women who have come out on top.

Don't forget to keep a record of the words and expressions that you have learnt, review your notes
from time to time and try to use new vocabulary items whenever possible.

Task 1: Put the words in each line of the box in order according to their size (the smallest first, the largest last). In each list there is one word that does not belong with the others.

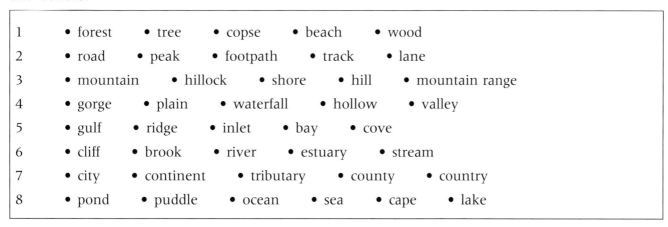

1	• forest	• tree	• copse	• beach	• wood
2	• road	• peak	• footpath	• track	• lane
3	• mountain	• hillock	• shore	• hill	• mountain range
4	• gorge	• plain	• waterfall	• hollow	• valley
5	• gulf	• ridge	• inlet	• bay	• cove
6	• cliff	• brook	• river	• estuary	• stream
7	• city	• continent	• tributary	• county	• country
8	• pond	• puddle	• ocean	• sea	• cape	• lake

Can you think of any examples of the following in your country?

Forest	
Mountain	
Mountain range	
Valley	
Gorge	
Plain	
Gulf	
River	
Estuary	
Sea	
Lake	

Task 2: Put the words and expressions in the box into their correct category in the tables below. Some can be included in more than one category.

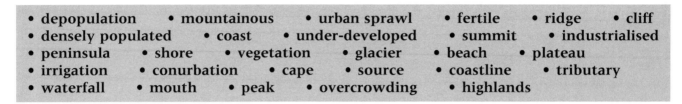

- depopulation • mountainous   • urban sprawl   • fertile   • ridge   • cliff
- densely populated   • coast   • under-developed   • summit   • industrialised
- peninsula   • shore   • vegetation   • glacier   • beach   • plateau
- irrigation   • conurbation   • cape   • source   • coastline   • tributary
- waterfall   • mouth   • peak   • overcrowding   • highlands

Geographical features associated with water and the sea	Geographical features associated with land, hills and mountains
Words associated with agriculture and rural land	**Words associated with towns and cities**

(*See also* Module 49: Town and country.)

Task 3: Now look at this report of a journey and fill in the gaps with one of the words or expressions from Tasks 1 and 2. In some cases, more than one answer may be possible. You may need to change some of the word forms.

We began our journey in the capital, Trinifuegos, a (1) . . . . conurbation of almost ten million. It is not a pretty place; heavily (2) . . . ., with huge factories belching out black fumes, and miles of (3) . . . . as housing estates and shopping centres spread out from the (4) . . . . centre for miles. It was a relief to leave.

As soon as we got into the countryside, things improved considerably. The climate is dry and it is difficult to grow anything, but thanks to (5) . . . ., which helps bring water in from the Rio Cauto (the huge river with its (6) . . . . high up in the snow-covered (7) . . . . of the Sierra Maestra (8) . . . .), the land is fertile enough to grow the sugar cane on which much of the economy is based. We saw few people, however, as many have moved to the towns and cities to look for more profitable work. It is largely due to this rural (9) . . . . that the sugar-cane industry is suffering.

Further south and we entered the Holguin (10) . . . . , with mountains rising high above us on both sides. The land here drops sharply to the sea and the slow-moving waters of the Rio Cauto give way to (11) . . . . which tumble over cliffs, and small, fast-moving (12) . . . . which are not even wide enough to take a boat. At this point, the road we were travelling along became a (13) . . . . which was only just wide enough for our vehicle, and then an unpaved (14) . . . . which almost shook the vehicle to pieces.

And then suddenly, the Pacific (15) . . . . was in front of us. Our destination was the town of Santiago de Gibara, built on a (16) . . . . sticking out into the blue waters. The countryside here undulates gently, with low (17) . . . . covered in rich tropical jungle. The open (18) . . . . surrounding the (19) . . . . of the Rio Cauto as it reaches the ocean is rich and (20) . . . . , ideal for growing the tobacco plants which need a lot of warm, damp soil.

That night, I lay in my cheap hotel, listening to the waves gently lapping the (21) . . . . , and when I eventually fell asleep, I dreamt of the people who had first inhabited this (22) . . . . almost two thousand years before.

53 Business and industry

Task 1: Look at sentences 1–16, and replace the words and expressions in **bold** with a word or expression in the box which has an opposite meaning.

> • unskilled labourers   • employees/workers/staff   • credit   • exports
> • loss   • demand for   • bust/recession   • shop floor   • state-owned industries
> • private   • expenditure   • lending   • net   • take on   • retail
> • white-collar

1 We have a limited **supply of** computer base units.

2 Last year, our company made a huge **profit**.

3 Our **gross** profits are up by almost 150% on last year.

4 Banks across the country are reporting a sharp drop in **borrowing**.

5 The company will **debit** your bank account with £528 each month.

6 The **wholesale** market has experienced a downturn since the recession began.

7 The government is encouraging short-term investors to put their money into the **public** sector.

8 **Private enterprises** are under a lot of financial pressure.

9 **Skilled workers** are demanding a 15% pay rise.

10 If this continues, we will have to **lay off** members of staff.

11 **Blue-collar** workers across the country are demanding improved working conditions.

12 He works for a company which **imports** camera equipment.

13 A lot of people have benefited from the recent **boom** in the electrical industry.

14 The **management** refuse to compromise on the quality of their products.

15 Overall **revenue** is down by almost 15%.

16 A fight broke out in the **boardroom** over terms and conditions of employment. (Note: you will have to change the preposition *in* to *on*.)

Task 2: Match the words and expressions in the first box with a dictionary definition from the list A–Q below.

> 1 automation   2 unemployment   3 inflation   4 balance of payments
> 5 taxation   6 GNP   7 interest rates   8 primary industries
> 9 secondary industries   10 service industries   11 nationalised industries
> 12 monopoly   13 output   14 income tax   15 VAT   16 deficit
> 17 key industries

A   The percentage charged for borrowing money. (**The Bank of England has raised . . . .**)

B   Industries involved in the manufacture of goods. (**. . . . . rely on a ready supply of raw materials.**)

C   The value of goods and services paid for in a country, including income earned in other countries. (**Last year's . . . . was close to £25 billion.**)

D   The amount which a firm, machine or person produces. (**The factory has doubled its . . . . in the last six months.**)

E   Industries involved in the production of raw materials. (**Coal mining is an important
. . . .**)

F   Installing machinery in place of workers (**. . . . . can be a mixed blessing – machines
usually tend to be out of order when you need them most.**)

G   Industries which do not make products but offer a service such as banking, insurance and
transport. (**. . . . . have become more important in the last decade.**)

H   The difference in value between a country's imports and exports. (**The government is trying to
reduce the . . . . deficit.**)

I   The amount by which expenditure is more than receipts in a firm's or country's accounts. (**The
company announced a two million pound . . . .**)

J   A system where one person or company supplies all of a product in one area without any
competition. (**The state has a . . . . of the tobacco trade.**)

K   Industries which were once privately owned, but now belong to the state. (**Workers in
. . . . are to get a 3% pay rise.**)

L   Lack of work. (**The figures for . . . . are rising.**)

M   The action of imposing taxes. (**Money raised by . . . . pays for all government
services.**)

N   The most important industries in a country. (**Oil is a . . . . which is essential to the
country's economy.**)

O   A state of economy where prices and wages are rising to keep pace with each other. (**The
government is trying to keep . . . . down below 3%.**)

P   A tax on money earned as wages or salary. (**She pays . . . . at the lowest rate.**)

Q   A tax imposed as a percentage of the invoice value of goods or services. An indirect tax.
(**. . . . . in Britain currently runs at 17.5%.**)

Task 3: Now look at this extract from a business programme and fill in the gaps with
one of the words or expressions from Tasks 1 and 2. In some cases, more than one
answer may be possible. You may need to change some of the word forms.

(1) . . . . rates are to rise by a further half a percent next month, putting further pressure on
homeowners paying mortgages. It will also discourage people from (2) . . . . money from the
high street banks, who are already under a lot of pressure. Last year, the National Bank was forced to
(3) . . . . 2,000 members of staff across the country, adding to the country's rapidly rising
rate of (4) . . . .

(5) . . . . rose in the last year by almost 6%, despite the government's pledge to keep price
and wage rises no higher than 3%. This has had a negative impact on (6) . . . . , since the
strong pound coupled with rising prices has made it almost impossible for foreign companies to buy
British goods and services. Especially affected are the (7) . . . . producing pharmaceuticals
and chemicals.

(8) . . . . workers in (9) . . . . industries across the country are demanding higher
(10) . . . . Unions and workers are negotiating with (11) . . . . chiefs for an eight
percent rise. This follows the announcement that the government want more investors to put their
money into the (12) . . . . sector.

(13) . . . . for home computers has finally overtaken the (14) . . . . , making it

once again a seller's market. There is now a two-week waiting list to receive a new computer. This has pushed prices up by almost a third.

Bradford Aerospace Technologies, where overall (15) . . . . for sales of aircraft parts has dropped by almost 10% in the last quarter, will shortly become a (16) . . . . industry in a final desperate attempt to keep it open. The government has promised it will keep on the current workforce.

Bad news too for Ranger Cars, who this week announced a (17) . . . . of almost five million pounds. A spokesman for the company blamed high labour costs and the reluctance by union leaders to approve increased (18) . . . . at the firm's factories. They insist that the installation of new machinery will lead to redundancies.

Don't forget to keep a record of the words and expressions that you have learnt, review your notes from time to time and try to use new vocabulary items whenever possible.

54 Global problems

Task 1: Complete sentences 1–15 with the correct word or expression from A, B or C. In each case two of the options are incorrectly spelt.

1 Thousands of buildings were flattened in the San Francisco . . . . of 1906.
   A. earthquack   **B. earthquake**   **C. earthquaik**

2 The . . . . damaged properties all along the coast.
   A. hurricane   **B. hurriccane**   **C. huriccane**

3 A . . . . struck the southern coast with tremendous force.
   A. tornadoe   **B. tornado**   **C. tornaddo**

4 The . . . . caused immense damage in the regions along the coast.
   A. taifun   **B. typhone**   **C. typhoon**

5 The . . . . has been dormant for years, but last month it showed signs of new life.
   A. volcano   **B. vulcano**   **C. volcanoe**

6 Several . . . . were heard during the night as the army occupied the city.
   A. explossions   **B. explosiones**   **C. explosions**

7 The American . . . . of 1861–1865 was fought between the south and the north.
   A. civil war   **B. sivil war**   **C. civvil war**

8 There has been a major . . . . on the motorway.
   A. acident   **B. accident**   **C. acciddent**

9 . . . . rain has brought serious problems.
   A. Torrential   **B. Torential**   **C. Torrantial**

10 The storm caused widespread . . . . along the coast.
   A. devvastation   **B. devustation**   **C. devastation**

11 The . . . . were caused by heavy rain.
   A. floodes   **B. floods**   **C. flouds**

12 Relief workers are bringing food to . . . . -stricken areas.
   A. draught   **B. drought**   **C. drouhgt**

13 . . . . is widespread in parts of Africa, with millions suffering from malnutrition.
   A. Famine   **B. Fammine**   **C. Faminne**

14 The authorities are taking steps to prevent an . . . . of cholera.
   A. epidemmic   **B. epidemic**   **C. eppidemic**

15 The . . . . was spread from rats to fleas and then on to humans.
   A. plague   **B. plaque**   **C. plaigue**

Task 2: Complete sentences 1–10 with an appropriate word or expression from the box. In some cases, more than one answer is possible. There are five words which do not fit into any of the sentences.

• disaster	• survivors	• spouted	• suffering	• ran	• erupted
• broke out	• shook	• casualties	• spread	• refugees	• relief
• flamed	• wobbled	• swept			

1 The disease . . . . rapidly, killing everybody in its path.
2 The fire . . . . through the slums, destroying everything.

3 When the volcano . . . . , people panicked and tried to escape.

4 The ground . . . . violently when the earthquake began.

5 Fierce fighting . . . . between government soldiers and rebel forces.

6 A funeral was held for the . . . . of the fire.

7 An aid convoy was sent to help . . . . of the hurricane.

8 . . . . from the conflict in Mantagua have been fleeing across the border.

9 The poor people in the city have experienced terrible . . . . as a result of the disaster.

10 International aid agencies are trying to bring . . . . to the starving population.

Task 3: Now look at this report and fill in the gaps with one of the words or expressions from Tasks 1 and 2. In some cases, more than one answer may be possible. You may need to change some of the word forms.

REPORT FROM THE INTERNATIONAL CHARITIES SUPPORT FOUNDATION (ICSF)

The last year has been a particularly busy one for the ICSF. Outlined below are a few of the areas we have been busy in.

1 Following (1) . . . . rain in eastern Mozamlumbi in January, millions were made homeless as (2) . . . . waters rose. The water also became polluted and there was a cholera (3) . . . . as people continued to use it for drinking and cooking. Furthermore, as the harvest had been destroyed and there was not enough food to go round, (4) . . . . became a problem. Charities around the world worked particularly hard to bring (5) . . . . to the area.

2 Mount Etsuvius, the (6) . . . . which had been dormant since 1968, (7) . . . . suddenly in April. Thousands had to be evacuated to camps thirty miles from the disaster area. They still have not been rehoused.

3 The (8) . . . . in the Caribbean in July, which saw wind speeds of up to 180 miles per hour, caused immense (9) . . . . on many islands. Islands off the Japanese coast also suffered their worst (10) . . . . in almost thirty years, with prolonged winds in excess of 150 miles per hour. There were many (11) . . . . who had to be evacuated to hospitals which were not properly equipped to deal with the disasters.

4 The (12) . . . . in the northern part of Somopia continued into its second year, with millions of acres of crops destroyed by lack of rain. Meanwhile, the (13) . . . . between those loyal to the president and those supporting the rebel leader continued into its fifth year. (14) . . . . from the conflict have been fleeing across the border, with stories of atrocities committed by both sides.

5 In October, a fire (15) . . . . through Londum, the ancient capital of Perania. The (16) . . . . , which probably started in a bakery, destroyed thousands of homes. There were several (17) . . . . when the fire reached a fireworks factory, and a number of people were killed.

6 An outbreak of bubonic (18) . . . . was reported in the eastern provinces of Indocuba in November. It is believed to have been caused by a sudden increase in the number of rats breeding in the sewers.

A full report will be available in February, and will be presented to the appropriate departments of the United Nations shortly afterwards.

Answers

Page 51: Condition answers

A:
1 You can borrow my dictionary **providing that** you return it before you go home. (We can also say *provided that*.)
2 You can't go to university **unless** you have good grades. (*Unless* means the same as *If you don't*.)
3 Pollution will get worse **as long as** we continue to live in a throwaway society. (We can also say *so long as*, although this is slightly more formal.)
4 Many developed countries are willing to waive the Third World debt **on condition that** the money is reinvested in education and medicine.
5 Some countries will never be able to rectify their deficits, **no matter how** hard they work. (Note word changes and sentence ending.)
6 Computers are difficult things to understand, **however many** books you read about them. (*However* is used in the same way as *no matter*.)
7 Crime is a problem, **wherever** you go.
On condition that is the most formal expression, and is generally stronger than the other words and expressions.

B: (We put the conditional clause at the beginning of a sentence if we consider it to be the most important part of the sentence.)
1 **Providing that** you return it before you go home, you can borrow my dictionary.
2 **Unless** you have good grades, you can't go to university.
3 **As long as** we continue to live in a throwaway society, pollution will get worse.
4 **On condition that** the money is reinvested in education and medicine, many developed countries are willing to waive the Third World debt.
5 **No matter how** hard they work, some countries will never be able to rectify their deficits.
6 **However many** books you read about them, computers are difficult things to understand.
7 **Wherever** you go, crime is a problem.

C: Form your own ideas.

D: 1. prerequisites   2. conditions   3. requirement

Page 52: Changes answers

1. adapt   2. adjust   3. transform   4. switch   5. alter   6. vary
7. exchange   8. expand   9. increase   10. dissolve   11. swell   12. disappear
13. renew   14. renovate   15. promote (in the second sentence, *promote* means to make sure people know about something by advertising it)   16. demote   17. fade   18. replace   19. cure (in the second sentence, *cure* means to preserve meat or fish by putting it in salt)   20. reduce
   Other words and expressions which you might find useful include:

• swap/shrink/melt/grow/heal/decline/enlarge/downsize/take to something

Page 54: Describing and analysing tables answers

A: 1. Cilicia + Cappadocia   2. Cappadocia   3. Lycia   4. Moesia   5. Cappadocia
6. Moesia   7. Lycia   8. Moesia   9. Moesia   10. Lycia   11. Lycia
12. Cilicia   13. Cappadocia

> The verbs *rise* and *increase* have the same meaning here. We can also say *climb*. These verbs can also be nouns.
>   The verbs *fall*, *drop* and *decline* have the same meaning here. These verbs can also be nouns.
>   The adverbs *steadily* and *noticeably* can have the same meaning here. They can also be adjectives (*steady*, *noticeable*).
>   The adverbs *sharply*, *rapidly* and *dramatically* can have the same meaning here. They can also be adjectives (*sharp*, *rapid*, *dramatic*).

B: Suggested answers:

1 The number of people employed in industry rose/increased steadily/noticeably between 1996 and 2000/over the five year period.
  or
  There was a steady/noticeable rise/increase in the number of people employed in industry between 1996 and 2000/over the five-year period.

2 The number of people employed in retail rose/increased slightly between 1996 and 2000/over the five-year period.
  or
  There was a slight rise/increase in the number of people employed in retail between 1996 and 2000/over the five year period.

3 The number of people employed in public services remained constant between 1999 and 2000.
  or
  There was a constant level of people employed in public services between 1999 and 2000.

4 The number of people employed in tourism fell/dropped/declined between 1996 and 1998, but rose/increased in 1999 and 2000.
  or
  There was a fall/drop/decline in the number of people employed in tourism between 1996 and 1998 and then a rise/increase in 1999 and 2000.

5 The number of unemployed between 1998 and 2000 remained constant.
  or
  There was a constant level of unemployment 1998 and 2000.

6 There was a considerable discrepancy between those employed in industry and those working in retail in 1996.

7 The number of people employed in industry rose/increased slightly between 1998 and 1999.
  or
  There was a slight rise/increase in the number of people employed in industry between 1998 and 1999.

Other words and expressions which you might find useful include:

- for things going up: rocket/jump/edge up/soar/creep up/peak (especially for numbers, prices, etc.)
- for things going down: slump/plunge/slip back/slip down/plummet/drop/bottom out (especially when talking about prices)

Page 56: How something works answers

1. thermostat (a heat controlling device in, e.g. a kettle or electric heater)   2. compact disc player   3. aerosol
4. aeroplane (USA = airplane)   5. camera   6. food processor   7. firework
  The other words in the grid are:

- Kettle/computer/car engine/television/toaster/microwave oven/ballpoint pen/lightbulb/bicycle

Other words and expressions you might find useful include:

- Reflects/turns/starts/stops/records/turns up/turns down/winds/unwinds/revolves/folds/unfolds/reverses

Note: When we describe how an object works and there is no person or other agent involved in our description, we use the *active voice* ('Light *enters* the glass object and a small door opens up'). When there is a person involved in the process, we usually use the *passive voice* ('This *can be released* . . .'; '. . . a button *is pressed*'). This is because the action or process is more important than the person doing it.

Page 57: Writing a letter answers

A: 1. B (the most acceptable beginning in British formal letters)   2. A   3. C (*I would like to . . .* is a common way of beginning a letter in many situations, e.g. complaining, applying for a job, asking for information. It is also possible to say *I am writing to . . .*)   4. C   5. A   6. C   7. A (we can also say *Thank you for your attention **to** this matter*)   8. C (we can also use *I refer* to letters and phone calls you have received: *I refer to your call of 12 March*)   9. B   10. B (*Best wishes* is used with more informal letters)   11. A

B: 1. False. Formal letters should be as brief and to the point as possible.   2. False.   3. False   4. False. It is not necessary to include your name   5. True (In some countries, writing abbreviated dates could be confusing. In Britain, 1/4/00 is the 1 April. In the USA it is the 4 January.)   6. True   7. False (A letter which is not broken into paragraphs can be difficult and confusing to read. You should have at least three paragraphs: Paragraph 1: explaining why you are writing. Paragraph 2+: details. Final paragraph: action to be taken – e.g. 'I look forward to hearing from you soon'.)

Page 59: Presenting an argument answers

A: The best order is: 1. A   2. H   3. K   4. M   5. E   6. G   7. B
8. J   9. F   10. O   11. C   12. N   13. L   14. D   15. I   16. P
   When you are asked to present an argument, you should always look at it from two sides, giving reasons why you agree and disagree before reaching a conclusion.
   Other words and expressions which you might find useful include:

• I believe that/despite this/in spite of this/also/thirdly/I think/finally/in conclusion/nonetheless/admittedly/on the contrary/at any rate/notwithstanding/for all that/even if

Page 60: Location answers

A: 1. parallel to/in close proximity to (we can also say *near to/close to*)   2. surrounded by   3. on the left-hand side of   4. in the bottom left-hand corner of   5. directly opposite   6. halfway between (we can also say *midway between*)   7. exactly in the middle of   8. roughly in the middle of   9. at the top of
10. in the top left-hand corner of   11. to the left of/in close proximity to   12. at right angles to/perpendicular to
13. to the right of/in close proximity to   14. in the top right-hand corner of   15. at the bottom of
16. in close proximity to   17. on the right-hand side of   18. in the bottom right-hand corner of
19. stands outside
   Other words and expressions which you might find useful include:

• in the north – south – east – west of/to the north – south – east – west of/on the corner (of a street)/on the other side of/approximately/in front of/behind/across from/above/below/beneath/beside

Page 62: Contrast and comparison answers

1. A   2. B   3. B   4. C (*differentiate* and *distinguish* have exactly the same meaning)
5. C   6. A   7. C   8. A   9. B   10. C   11. A   12. C   13. C
14. B   15. B

Page 63: Joining/becoming part of something bigger answers

Verbs: 1. linked   2. amalgamated/merged   3. blended   4. merged/amalgamated
5. incorporated   6. integrated/assimilated   7. assimilated/integrated   8. swallowed up/took over
9. got together   10. took over/swallowed up (*swallowed up* is less formal than *took over*)
Nouns: 1. alliance   2. union   3. federation   4. alloy   5. compound
6. synthesis   7. unification   8. blend   9. coalition   10. merger

Page 64: Reason and result answers

A: 1. The police asked him his reason for speeding through the town.   2. He failed his exam due to/on account of/ owing to (these expressions have the same meaning as *because of*) his lack of revision.   3. A persistent cough prompted him to seek professional medical help.   4. She started haranguing the crowd with the aim of starting a riot.   5. He spent the whole weekend revising in order to pass his exams.   6. They came in quietly so as not to wake anyone.   7. He refused to lend anyone money on the grounds that people rarely repay a loan.   8. The bank manager refused to lend the company more money on account of/due to/owing to its low turnover and poor sales history.   9. The school was forced to close due to/on account of/owing to poor student attendance.   10. What were your motives in upsetting me like that?   11. What are the effects of a large earthquake?   12. Stress and overwork can affect different people in different ways.   13. The army attacked without considering the consequences of/effects of its action.   14. He failed to send off his application form and as a consequence was unable to enrol for the course.   15. Riots and street fighting ensued when the police officers on trial were acquitted.

B: 1. ensued   2. consequences of/effects of   3. in order to   4. with the aim of   5. on account of/due to/owing to   6. reason for   7. prompted him to   8. on the grounds that   9. so as not to   10. affect

Page 65: Generalisations and specifics answers

A: 1. D   2. A   3. B   4. H   5. L   6. E   7. O   8. F   9. I
10. J   11. N   12. M   13. G   14. C   15. K

B:

- General things: outline/generalisations/gist/in general
- Specific things: specifies/technicality/peculiar to/details/itemise/minutiae/characteristics/illustration/illustrate/exemplifies/ peculiarity
- Other words and expressions you might find useful include: on the whole/for the most part/generalities/general terms/to generalise/list (as a verb)/specify

Page 67: Focusing attention answers

A: 1. simply   2. largely   3. primarily   4. mainly   5. exclusively   6. particularly
7. specifically   8. notably   9. mostly   10. purely   11. chiefly
The word in the shaded vertical strip is **principally**

B:

- Only or solely: simply/exclusively/specifically/purely
- In most cases, normally or the main reason: largely/primarily/mainly/particularly/notably/mostly/chiefly

Other words and expressions you might find useful include:

- for the simple reason that/purely on account of

Page 69: Opinion, attitude and belief answers

A: 1. opinion   2. concerned   3. convinced   4. regarding   5. disapproval   6. maintains
7. reckon (an informal word which means *think* or *believe*)   8. suspect   9. doubt   10. disapprove
11. exception   12. fanatical   13. obsessive (Note: obsessive *about*/obsessed *with*)   14. moderates
15. conservative   16. committed   17. dedicated   18. traditional

B:

- Political beliefs: a republican/a revolutionary/left-wing/right-wing/a socialist/a royalist/a conservative/a liberal/a communist/ a fascist/middle-of-the-road/an anarchist
- Personal convictions and philosophies: opinionated/pragmatic/a Muslim/an intellectual/tolerant/a moralist/narrow-minded/ bigoted/open-minded/a vegan/a Buddhist/a vegetarian/dogmatic/moral/religious/a Hindu/a stoic

Other words and expressions you might find useful include:

- view (as a verb)/attitude/protest/condemn/object to something/condemnation/denounce/revulsion/disparage/scornful/ applaud/agree with/disagree with/disagreement/hold the view that/from my point of view/for and – or against

Page 71: Stopping something answers

1. delete   2. repeal   3. deter   4. dissuade   5. rescind   6. suppress   7. sever (we can also use the expression *break off*)   8. turn down (we can also say *reject* or *decline*)   9. back out (we can also say *withdraw*)   10. deny   11. cancel   12. quash   13. give up   14. put an end to   15. remove (less formally, we can also say *strike*, but only if we are referring to something on paper, e.g. *'Strike his name from the list'*)

Other words and expressions you might find useful include:

- discard/refuse/clamp down on somebody – something/delay (to stop something temporarily)

Page 72: Objects and actions answers

A: 1. rotate   2. spin   3. revolve   4. slide   5. subside   6. evaporate   7. congeal (for blood, we use the word *clot*)   8. flow   9. freeze   10. melt   11. wobble   12. escape (we can also say *leak*)   13. bounce   14. vibrate   15. grow   16. fade   17. rise
18. set   19. turn   20. change   21. erode   22. spread   23. meander   24. burn
25. smoulder   26. crumble   27. expand   28. contract   29. stretch   30. crack
31. spill   32. explode   33. ring   34. sink   35. float   36. erupt   37. trickle

Note: Several of these verbs can also be nouns, and in many cases the meaning of the word changes. Compare, for example, *a contract* and *to contract*.

B: 1. stretched   2. exploded   3. float   4. rising   5. fade   6. cracked
7. subsided   8. revolved   9. set   10. slid

Other words and expressions you might find useful include:

- move/run/stop/fall down/come in/get up/break/bend/dance/cool/solidify/thaw/trickle/drench

See also Module 4: How something works

Page 74: Likes and dislikes answers

A:

- Positive connotations: yearn for/passionate about/fond of/captivated by/fancy/keen on/look forward to/long for/appeal to/attracted to/fascinated by/tempted by
- Negative connotations: loathe/dread/detest/cannot stand/repel/disgust/revolt/cannot bear

B: 1. A + B = ✓   2. A = ✓ B = ✗   3. A = ✗ B = ✓   4. A = ✗ B = ✓   5. A + B = ✓
6. A = ✗ B = ✓   7. A = ✗ B = ✓   8. A = ✓ B = ✗   9. A + B = ✓   10. A = ✓ B = ✗
11. A = ✗ B = ✓   12. A = ✗ B = ✓   13. A = ✓ B = ✗   14. A + B = ✓   15. A + B = ✓
16. A + B = ✓   17. A + B = ✓   18. A + B = ✓   19. A + B = ✓   20. A = ✗ B = ✓

Page 76: Time answers

A:

- Part 1: 1. Prior to (this expression is usually followed by a noun or by an -ing verb: For example: *Prior to visiting the country, he had to study the language*) 2. By the time 3. Formerly/Previously 4. precede 5. Previously 6. Previously/Earlier
- Part 2: 1. While/As/Just as (*While* is usually used to talk about long actions. *When* is usually used to talk about short actions) 2. During/Throughout (*During* must always be followed by a noun. *Throughout* can be used on its own. For example: *The concert was boring and I slept throughout*) 3. In the meantime/Meanwhile (If these words are followed by another word, that word must be a noun) 4. At that very moment
- Part 3. 1. Following (This word is always followed by a noun. We can also say *after*) 2. As soon as/Once/The minute that (These words and expressions are always followed by an action) 3. Afterwards

B:

- (1 – the past): in medieval times/back in the 1990s/in those days/a few decades ago/at the turn of the century/in my childhood/youth/last century/from 1996 to 1998
- (2 – the past leading to the present): ever since/over the past six weeks/lately/for the past few months
- (3 – the present): as things stand/nowadays/at this moment in time/at this point in history/these days
- (4 – the future): for the next few weeks/one day/from now on/over the coming weeks and months/in another five years' time/by the end of this year/for the foreseeable future/sooner or later

Page 78: Obligation and option answers

A: 1. False (you must take your own pencil and eraser) 2. True 3. False (he had to pay the money back) 4. False (they don't have to pay any income tax at all) 5. True 6. False (the doctors made him stop smoking) 7. True 8. False (you can attend the classes if you want to) 9. False (you must wear a crash helmet. We can also use the word *obligatory*) 10. True.

B: 1. obliged/required 2. no alternative 3. liable for 4. compulsory 5. voluntary 6. mandatory 7. required 8. forced 9. optional 10. exempt

Page 79: Success and failure answers

A:
1 The two warring countries managed to **reach/achieve** a *compromise* over the terms for peace.
2 During his first year as President he managed to **achieve/accomplish/fulfil** *a lot more* than his predecessor had in the previous five.
3 The company couldn't afford to move to new premises but were able to **reach/secure** *an agreement* for a new lease.
4 He worked hard at his job and was soon able to **achieve/realise/fulfil** his *ambitions* of being promoted to marketing manager. (Note: *realise* can also be written *realize*)
5 The country badly needed to increase its overall standard of living and attempted to **achieve/reach/attain** its *targets* – those of free education and healthcare – within eight years.
6 After four years of hard work, the motor racing team managed to **achieve/realise** their *dreams* of winning the Monaco Grand Prix.
7 He desperately wanted to start a new job, but first of all he had to **fulfil** his *obligations* to his current employer.
8 Many people want to be rich, but few **achieve/realise/fulfil** their *goal* of becoming millionaires.
9 I have a lot of plans, and one of them is to **achieve/realise/fulfil** my *aims* of doing well at school and then going to university.

Note: Instead of *manage to* (+ the infinitive form of the verb), we can say *succeed in* (+ the –ing form of the verb). Example: He *managed to pass* his exam/He *succeeded in passing* his exam.

B: 1. B   2. A   3. B   4. C   5. B   6. C (we can also say *backfired*, when a plan turns out exactly the opposite to what was expected. For example: *All their holiday plans backfired when the children got chicken pox*) Other words and expressions which you might find useful include:

- come off (an informal expression meaning *to succeed*)/fail/come to nothing

Page 81: Ownership, giving, lending and borrowing answers

A: 1. landlords (*landlady* = female. We can also use the word *landowner*)   2. owners/proprietors 3. owners   4. property   5. estate   6. possessions   7. belongings (*possessions* usually refers to **everything** we own – for example, our homes, furniture, etc. *Belongings* usually refers to **smaller things** – for example, a coat, a briefcase, etc.)   8. lease   9. loan   10. mortgage   11. tenants   12. rent/mortgage 13. donation (we can also say *contribution*) Note: These words can be either *nouns* or *verbs*: lease/rent/mortgage/loan. *Loan* can also be used as an adjective, e.g. *a loan shark*.

B: 1. lend   2. rent   3. hire   4. borrow   5. contribute (we can also say *donate*) 6. provide for   7. leave   8. allocate/provide   9. provide Other words and expressions which you might find useful include:

- supply (somebody) with (something)/cater for/present (somebody) with (something)

Page 83: Around the world answers

A: 1. C   2. B (*Antarctica* is the name of the continent and is not preceded by *the*)   3. B   4. A 5. C (countries between North and South America, i.e., south of Mexico and north of Colombia)   6. A (all countries south of the USA where Spanish or Portuguese is widely spoken as a first language)   7. C   8. C 9. C (*Mainland* Europe and *Continental* Europe have the same meaning. British and Irish people often refer to Continental Europe as *the Continent*)   10. B   11. C

B:

-ese (e.g. China = Chinese)	-(i)an (e.g. Brazil = Brazilian)	-ish (e.g. Britain = British)	-i (e.g. Pakistan = Pakistani)	-ic (e.g. Iceland = Icelandic)	Others (e.g. France = French)
Portuguese Lebanese Japanese Burmese Maltese	Belgian Malaysian (we can also say *Malay*) Norwegian Peruvian Russian Iranian American Canadian Australian	Irish Finnish English Scottish Swedish Spanish Turkish Danish Polish	Bangladeshi Israeli Kuwaiti Yemeni Iraqi	Arabic (Adjectives with – *ic* are usually used to talk about racial groups rather than nationalities. For example, *Slavic, Nordic*, etc.)	Greek Welsh Dutch Thai Swiss Filipino

C: 1. a dialect   2. Your mother tongue is the language you first learned to speak as a child and which you continue to use at home, with your friends, your family, etc.   3. bilingual/multilingual   4. The seven continents are: Europe/North America/South America/Asia/Australasia/Africa/Antarctica. In some countries, more than one language is officially spoken (for example, in Belgium some people speak French and some speak Flemish)

Page 85: Groups answers

A:

People in general	People working together	Animals	Objects
huddle	company	litter	batch
throng	team	swarm	heap/pile
gang	platoon	flock	stack
crowd	staff	herd	bundle
group	crew	pack	bunch
	cast	shoal/school	set

B: 1. crowd/throng   2. huddle/group   3. set   4. staff   5. company   6. herd
7. batch   8. gang/crowd   9. cast   10. heap/pile   11. group   12. shoal
13. litter   14. crew   15. flock   16. team   17. throng/crowd   18. platoon
19. bundle   20. bunch   21. stack   22. pack   23. swarm

C: A. lecture   B. delegation   C. tutorial   D. symposium   E. seminar   F. tribunal

Page 87: Shape and features answers

A: 1. E   2. D   3. J   4. F   5. A   6. L   7. G   8. H   9. I
10. K   11. B   12. C

B: 1. B   2. A   3. C   4. C   5. A   6. C   7. A   8. C

C: 1. D   2. F   3. H   4. G   5. I   6. B   7. E   8. A   9. C

Page 89: Size, quantity and dimension answers

A:

- Big: 3   4   5   6   7   9   10   11   12   14
  15   16   17   18   19   20   22   23   24   25
- Small: 1 (note the pronunciation:/maɪ'njuːt/)   2   8   13   21

B: 1. a long-distance journey   2. a great deal of time   3. dozens of times   4. A minute amount of dust
5. a gigantic wave   6. a huge waste of time   7. a colossal statue   8. plenty of food
9. A broad river   10. A vast crowd of supporters   11. a gargantuan meal/plenty of food
12. a giant building/a vast room   13. a mammoth job/tons of work (both these expressions are informal)
14. a deep lake   15. a minuscule piece of cloth   16. an enormous book
17. a mammoth job/tons of work   18. a high mountain   19. a monumental error
20. a tiny car   21. a giant building   22. wide avenue   23. a shallow pool   24. a tall man
25. A narrow alleyway

Page 91: Emphasis and misunderstanding answers

A: 1. F   2. B   3. E   4. C   5. A   6. D

B: 1. emphasise/accentuate   2. prominent   3. emphasis/accent/stress   4. emphasised/accentuated/stressed
5. put great stress   6. of crucial importance/extremely important   7. emphasis

C: 1. confused   2. confusion   3. mix-up (informal. It can also be a verb: *to mix up*)   4. obscure
5. distorted   6. impression/misapprehension   7. assumed   8. mistaken
9. impression/misapprehension
Note: Word forms.

Verb	Noun	Adjective	Adverb
confuse	confusion	confusing/confused	confusingly
distort	distortion	distorted	
misapprehend	misapprehension		
mistake	mistake	mistaken	mistakenly
assume	assumption		

Page 93: Changes answers

A: 1. True   2. True   3. False: there has been an *improvement*   4. False: there has been an *increase*   5. False: there has been a *strengthening* of the dollar   6. False: there has been a *relaxation* of border *controls*   7. False: we're *increasing* or *building up* our stocks of coal   8. True   9. False: there has been a *slight* fall   10. False: they're going to *decrease* the number   11. False: there has been a *decline*
12. False: there has been a *tightening up* of the rules   13. False: there has been a *widening* of the gap
14. True   15. False: there has been a *downward* trend   16. True   17. True   18. True
19. True   20. False: British people want to *broaden* their horizons
   Most of the words in this task can be *verbs* as well as *nouns*. Use a dictionary to check which ones.
   Other words and expressions which you might find useful include:

• raise/lower/shrink/extend/introduce/enlarge/drop in/ability/open/close/lessen/heighten/lower/deepen/stretch/extend/
  spread/widen/shorten

See also Module 3: Describing and analysing tables

Page 95: Opposites answers

• Verbs: 1. rejected   2. denied   3. retreated   4. refused   5. defended
  6. demolished   7. simplified   8. abandoned   9. withdrew   10. deteriorated
  11. refused (to let)   12. rewarded   13. lowered   14. set
  15. fell (we can also say *dropped*)   16. loosened

• Adjectives: 1. clear   2. easy   3. graceful   4. detrimental (we can also say *harmful*)
  5. approximate   6. innocent   7. even   8. scarce   9. flexible   10. clear
  11. crude (we can also say *primitive*)   12. delicate (we can also say *mild*)   13. dim
  14. compulsory (we can also say *obligatory*)   15. reluctant

Note: A lot of words have more than one opposite, depending on their meaning (for example, the opposites of *strong* are *weak/feeble* (if you are talking about **physical strength**), *delicate/mild* (if you are talking about **taste**), *dim/faint* (if you are talking about **light**) or just *weak* (if you are talking about the strength of a drink). Use a dictionary to check if you are not sure.

Page 97: Addition, equation and conclusion answers

A:

Addition (For example: and)	Equation (For example: equally)	Conclusion (For example: in conclusion)
along with as well as also too in addition besides what's more furthermore moreover along with (this could also go into the next box)	likewise similarly in the same way correspondingly	to sum up briefly it can be concluded that to conclude in brief thus to summarise therefore

B: 1. Furthermore/Moreover/In addition/What's more (this is less formal than the other expressions)
2. As well as/Besides   3. Likewise/Similarly/In the same way (the verbs in both sentences (i.e. *respect*) are the same and refer to the same thing, so we can use a word of equation here)   4. As well as/Along with
5. In addition   6. Likewise/Similarly   7. Likewise/In the same way/Correspondingly
8. In brief   9. It can be concluded that   10. Therefore (*To sum up*, *to conclude* and *to summarise* are usually used to conclude longer pieces of writing. *Thus* is slightly more formal than *therefore*, but has the same meaning)
    Note: It is important that you are familiar with the way these words and expressions are used, including the other words in a sentence that they 'work' with. Use a dictionary to look up examples of these words and expressions, and keep a record of them that you can refer to the next time you use them.

Page 99: Task commands answer

1. N   2. I   3. R   4. L   5. E   6. P   7. F   8. K   9. G
10. R   11. J   12. N   13. Q   14. C   15. O   16. H   17. B
18. A   19. M   20. D
Other words and expressions which you might find useful include:

- give an account of/calculate/characterise/classify/comment on/consider/contrast/criticize/deduce/describe/determine/differentiate between/distinguish between/elucidate/enumerate/express/list/mention/relate/show/speculate/state

Page 101: Confusing words and false friend answers

1. action/activity   2. advise/advice   3. effect/affect   4. appreciable/appreciative
5. assumption/presumption   6. prevent/avoid   7. beside/besides   8. shortly/briefly
9. channel/canal   10. conscious/conscientious   11. continuous/continual   12. inspect/control

13. objections/criticism   14. injury/damage/harm   15. invent/discover   16. for/during/while
17. However/Moreover   18. inconsiderable/inconsiderate   19. intolerable/intolerant   20. job/work
21. lies/lay   22. watch/look at   23. permit/permission   24. possibility/chance
25. practise/practice   26. priceless/worthless (we can also say valueless)   27. principle/principal/principal/principle
28. procession/process   29. rise/raise   30. respectful/respectable   31. treat/cure

Note: some of these words have more than one meaning. For example, a *television* **channel** and a **channel** *of water between two land masses.* Use a dictionary to check for other meanings.

Other confusing words/false friends include:

- actually – now/already – yet/afraid of – worried about/bring – fetch/conduct – direct/consequences – sequences/driver – chauffeur/formidable – wonderful/fun – funny/go – play (for sports and games)/come along with – follow/kind – sympathetic/lend – borrow/nature – countryside/overcome – overtake/pass – take (an exam)/recipe – receipt/remember – remind/scenery – view/sensible – sensitive/special – especially/take – bring

Page 104: Useful interview expressions answers

Agreeing with somebody:	13	17	18	23	26	30
Disagreeing with somebody:	10 (followed by your opinion) (followed by your opinion)		11 29	16 33 (slightly more forceful)	19	24
Interrupting:	9 28 35 (You shouldn't interrupt too often. In any case, during the interview the examiner will leave you to do most of the talking)					
Asking for clarification or repetition:	6	12	22	32	36 (Don't just say *What?* Or *Eh?*)	
Asking somebody for their opinion:	5	14	37			
Saying something in another way:	3 8 20 for summing up)	21	25	27 (this can also be used		
Giving yourself time to think:	1	7	21	34		
Summing up:	2	4	15	31		

Page 109: Spelling answers

A:

1 advise = advice

Many English words can be nouns *and* verbs without a change in spelling. However, some words which end in **-ice** when they are nouns end with **-ise** when they become verbs. For example, practi**c**e (noun) = practi**s**e (verb)

2 acheive = achieve

A lot of English words use a combination of **i** and **e**. The order of these letters can be confusing

In most words where these letters are pronounced as *ee* (as in cheese), the **i** comes before the **e** (for example, s**ie**ge, th**ie**f, f**ie**ld, bel**ie**f, p**ie**ce) unless the letters are preceded by the letter *c* (for example, c**ei**ling, conc**ei**t, rec**ei**ve, dec**ei**ve)

However, not all words follow this rule. Exceptions include *caffeine, protein, neither, either* and *seize*

When the letters are pronounced *ay* (as in hate), the **e** comes before the **i** (for example, w**ei**gh, v**ei**l, n**ei**ghbour, **ei**ght)

There are other words which must be learned individually. These are: foreign, forfeit, height, heir, leisure, their, surfeit, sovereign

3 aquire = acquire

A lot of English words contain silent letters – in other words, a letter which we do not pronounce when we say the word
There are very few rules to tell you which is which, so you must learn each word individually or use a dictionary to check the spelling of a word if you are not sure

Some common examples of silent letters include:

Silent A: Febru**a**ry, parli**a**ment, marri**a**ge

Silent B: com**b**, bom**b**, wom**b**, dou**b**t

Silent C: cons**c**ience, s**c**ene, dis**c**ipline, s**c**issors

Silent D: We**d**nesday, han**d**some

Silent G: campai**g**n, desi**g**n

Silent H: g**h**ost, sc**h**ool, ve**h**icle, r**h**ythm

Silent I: bus**i**ness, hyg**i**ene, nu**i**sance

Silent N: autum**n**, colum**n**, condem**n**

Silent T: lis**t**en, mor**t**gage

Silent U: bisc**u**it, colleag**u**e (which also has a silent **e** at the end), g**u**arantee, g**u**ess

Silent W: ans**w**er, **w**hole

Silent GH: thou**gh**, thorou**gh**, wei**gh**, hei**gh**t

4 swimming = swimming
We double the last letter of single-syllable words ending with a single vowel and a single consonant when we add a suffix (e.g. **-ing**):

– swim – swimming, run – running, dip – dipped

We usually do the same thing if a two-syllable word is stressed on the second syllable:

– begin – beginning, regret – regrettable, prefer – preferring

We do not double the last letter in the following cases:

– when a word ends with **w**, **x** or **y**

– when the suffix begins with a consonant (e.g. bad – badly)

– when a word ends with **l** and the suffix **–ly** is added (e.g. playful – playfully)

– when two vowels come before the final consonant (e.g. weep – weeping)

5 thiefs = thieves
Most nouns are regular. This means that we add an **s** to make them plural (e.g. car – cars). However, some nouns are irregular – we either do not add an **s** to the word to make it plural or we add **s** plus some other letters

In nouns which end with a consonant and **y**, the **y** changes to **i** and we add **s**:

– party – parties, baby – babies, worry – worries

In nouns which end with **s**, **sh**, **tch** and **x**, we add **es**:

– bus – buses, dish – dishes, watch – watches, box – boxes

In some nouns which end in **f** or **fe**, we replace the **f** with a **v** and add **es**:

– calf – calves, half – halves, knife – knives, life – lives, wife – wives

In some words which end with **o**, we add **es**:

– cargo – cargoes, echo – echoes, hero – heroes

Some words do not change at all:

– fish, deer, sheep

And some words have their own individual rules:

– man – men, child – children, woman – women, person – people

6 hopeing = hoping
We drop the **e** from a word when a suffix which begins with a vowel (e.g. **-ing**) is added to a word which ends in a consonant plus a silent **e**:

– hope – hoping, tape – taping, give – giving, immature – immaturity

We also drop the **e** from a word when a suffix which begins with a vowel is added to a word which ends in a vowel plus a silent **e**:

– continue – continuity, pursue – pursuing, argue – arguable

When a suffix begins with a consonant (e.g. **-ment**) we do not usually drop the **e**, although there are some exceptions (e.g. awe – awful, true – truly)

7 happyness = happiness
   We change the **y** to **i** when it follows a consonant and a suffix is added (e.g. happy – happiness)

   We do not usually change the **y** to **i** when the **y** follows a vowel (e.g. play – playful) or when the suffix added is **–ing** (e.g. pry – prying)

B: 1. acknowledgment = acknowledgement   2. argueable = arguable   3. benefitting = benefiting
4. busness = business   5. campain = campaign   6. cancelations = cancellations
7. changeable = changeable   8. condeming = condemning   9. consientious = conscientious
10. hieght = height   11. managable = manageable   12. decieved = deceived   13. lifes = lives
14. survivers = survivors   15. practice = practise

C: 1. C   2. B   3. B   4. A   5. C   6. C   7. C   8. B   9. C
10. C   11. A

Page 111: Education answers

Task 1

1. A (we can also use the word *retake*)   2. B   3. B   4. C   5. C   6. A   7. C
8. B   9. B   10. C   11. B   12. A

The British higher education system is formed of universities and colleges, where students can take degrees in various specialised subjects. Students need a certain level of passes at 'A' levels to enter a university, and most universities ask students to come for special entrance exams and interviews. Fees in higher education are in some cases met by grants, but many students are required to pay for their tuition fees and take out loans to do this.

Task 2

1. kindergarten (we can also use the words *nursery* or *playschool*)   2. primary   3. skills/literacy/numeracy
4. secondary   5. discipline (this can also be a verb)/pass (the opposite of this is *fail*)   6. course (we can also use the word *programme*)   7. enrol   8. graduated (this can also be a noun – a *graduate*; a student who has finished a course at university. A student who is still at university is called an *undergraduate*)/degree
9. correspondence (we can also use the expression *distance learning*)   10. qualifications
11. evening class/day release

Task 3

1. skills   2 + 3. literacy/numeracy (in either order)   4. kindergarten   5. primary   6. secondary
7. discipline   8. pass   9. qualifications   10. acquire   11. health   12. further
13. enrol   14. higher   15. graduate   16. degree   17. higher   18. evening class
19. day release   20. correspondence   21. mature   22. opportunity
   Other words and expressions which you might find useful include:

• pupil power (a relatively new expression suggesting a school or college where the students are partly responsible for choosing what and how they learn)/faculty/subject/resources/campus/adult education/infant school/junior school/comprehensive school/take *or* sit an exam/private education/co-educational/lecture/seminar/tutorial

Page 113: The media answers

Task 1

1. E 2. H 3. C 4. B 5. A 6. D 7. L 8. F 9. I
10. M 11. J 12. K 13. G

In Britain, the most popular broadsheets include: The Guardian, The Independent, The Times, The Daily Telegraph and the Financial Times. The most popular tabloids include: The Sun, The Mirror, The Daily Mail and The Daily Express.

Task 2

1. freedom of the press 2. media tycoon (we can also use the expression *media mogul*)
3. censorship 4. unscrupulous 5. exploiting 6. invasion of privacy 7. paparazzi
8/9. information/entertainment (in either order) 10. chequebook journalism 11. libel
12. readership 13. gutter press

Task 3

1. broadsheets 2. coverage 3. current affairs 4. reporters 5. journalists
6. tabloids 7. broadcasts 8. Internet 9. websites 10. download
11/12. information/entertainment (in either order) 13. gutter press 14. invasion of privacy/chequebook
journalism 15. paparazzi 16. libel 17. chequebook journalism 18. unscrupulous
19. Internet/web 20. information overload 21. logging on 22. censorship
23. freedom of the press
    Other words and expressions which you might find useful include:

* *Types of television programme:* documentary/soap opera/quiz show/sitcom/drama/weather forecast/game show/variety show/commercial/chat show
* *Parts of a newspaper:* headline/editorial/advertisement/what's on/entertainment/colour supplement/fashion/business/financial/sport/horoscope
* state-controlled/journal/slander/tune in/read between the lines/downmarket/upmarket/upbeat

Page 115: Work answers

Task 1

1. ☺ 2. ☹ 3. ☺ 4. ☺ 5. ☹ 6. ☺ 7. ☹ 8. ☹ 9. ☹
10. ☹ 11. ☺ 12. ☹ 13. ☹ 14. ☹ 15. ☹ 16. ☺ 17. ☺
18. ☺ 19. ☹ 20. ☹ 21. ☹ 22. ☺ 23. ☹ (although some people enjoy a very demanding job)

'Sick Building Syndrome' is a recently discovered problem in which the design of a building adversely affects the people working in it. For example, in buildings with poor ventilation the employees often suffer from headaches or breathing problems.
    'Repetitive strain injury' (R.S.I.) is a pain in the arm or some other part of the body felt by someone who performs the same movement many times, such as when operating a computer keyboard.

Task 2

1. E   2. A   3. B   4. F   5. C   6. D

Task 3

1. employees   2. unskilled   3. semi-skilled   4. blue-collar   5. manufacturing industries   6. white-collar   7. service industries   8. job security   9. steady job   10. hiring   11. firing   12. stress   13. demanding   14. unsociable hours   15. repetitive strain injury   16. salary (a *salary* is paid monthly. We also use it to describe the amount of money an employee receives over a year: 'What is your salary?' '£24,000 a year/per annum.' We use the word *wage* or *wages* to describe money which is paid daily or weekly)   17. promotion   18. perks   19. incentive   20. increment (we can also use the expression *pay rise*)   21. sickness benefit   22. pension   23. self-employed

Other words and expressions which you might find useful include:

• employer/manual worker/profession/dismiss/dismissal/recruitment drive (when a company tries to employ a lot of new people)/overtime/fixed income/candidate/interview/interviewer/interviewee/leave (a formal word meaning *holiday*)

Page 117: Money and finance answers

Task 1

1 **Profit** is money you gain from selling something, which is more than the money you paid for it. **Loss** is money you have spent and not got back.
2 **Extravagant** describes somebody who spends a lot of money. **Frugal** or **economical** describes somebody who is careful with money.
3 A **current account** is a bank account from which you can take money at any time. A **deposit account** is a bank account which pays you interest if you leave money in it for some time (we can also use the expression *savings account* or *notice account*).
4 A **loan** is money which you borrow to buy something. A **mortgage** is a special kind of loan used to buy a house over a period of time.
5 To **deposit** money is to put money into a bank account. To **withdraw** money is to take money out of a bank account (*deposit* can be a noun or a verb. The noun form of *withdraw* is *withdrawal*).
6 A **wage** and a **salary** are money you receive for doing a job, but a wage is usually paid daily or weekly and a salary is usually paid monthly.
7 If you are **broke**, you have no money. It is an informal expression. If you are **bankrupt**, you are not able to pay back money you have borrowed. It is a very serious financial situation for somebody to be in.
8 In the UK, **shares** are one of the many equal parts into which a company's capital is divided. People who buy them are called *shareholders*. **Stocks** are shares which are issued by the government. **Dividends** are parts of a company's profits shared out among the shareholders.
9 **Income tax** is a tax on money earned as wages or salary. **Excise duty** is a tax on certain goods produced in a country, such as cigarettes or alcohol.
10 To **credit** somebody's bank account is to put money into the account. To **debit** somebody's bank account is to take money out. In the UK, many people pay for bills etc. using a system called *direct debit*, where money is taken directly from their account by the company providing the goods or service.
11 Traditionally a **bank** is a business organisation which keeps money for customers and pays it out on demand or lends them money, and a **building society** is more usually associated with saving money or lending people money to buy houses.
12 A **discount** is the percentage by which a full price is reduced to a buyer by the seller. A **refund** is money paid back when, for example, returning something to a shop. (It can also be a verb: *to refund*.)
13 A **bargain** is something bought more cheaply than usual (the word can have other meanings – check your dictionary). Something which is **overpriced** is too expensive. Something which is **exorbitant** costs much more than its true value.

14 A **worthless** object is something which has no value. A **priceless** object is an extremely valuable object.

15 If you **save** money, you put it to one side so that you can use it later. If you **invest** money, you put it into property, shares etc. so that it will increase in value.

16 **Inflation** is a state of economy where prices and wages increase. **Deflation** is a reduction of economic activity.

17 **Income** is the money you receive. **Expenditure** is the money you spend.

18 If you **lend** money, you let someone use your money for a certain period of time. If you **borrow** money from someone, you take money for a time, usually paying interest.

Task 2

1. F   2. I   3. L   4. E   5. J   6. K (the *Inland Revenue* is a British government department dealing with tax)   7. C   8. H   9. G   10. A   11. B   12. D

Task 3

1. borrow   2. loan   3. income   4. expenditure   5. overdraft   6. cost of living
7. Inflation   8. economise   9. building society   10. Interest   11. on credit
12. exorbitant   13. save   14. reductions   15. bargain   16. discount   17. invest
18. stocks   19. shares
   Other words and expressions which you might find useful include:

• Cash/cheque/credit card/statement/overdrawn/receipt/customs/inheritance tax/corporation tax/disability allowance/social security/currency/rate of exchange/investment/wealthy/debt/upwardly or downwardly mobile/equity/negative equity

Page 120: Politics answers

Task 1

1. democracy   2. independence (the adjective is independent)   3. candidate   4. totalitarian
5. authoritarian   6. technocrats   7. opposition   8. republic   9. sanctions   10. House
11. ideology   12. Parliament
   The word in the shaded vertical strip is 'dictatorship'.

The British Parliament is divided into two houses. These are:
1   The House of Commons. This is the lower house, which is made up of 659 elected members who are known as Members of Parliament, or MPs.
2   The House of Lords. This is the upper chamber, which is made up of hereditary peers or specially appointed men and women.
The House of Commons is the most important house. Many people in Britain want the House of Lords abolished because they see it as an outdated institution.

Task 2

1   False. It is a system of government with an *hereditary* king or queen.
2   False. A politician is a person who works for the *government*.
3   False. A statesman or stateswoman is an important *political* leader or representative of a country.
4   True
5   True.
6   False. A ministry is a government department.
7   True.

8 False. A policy is a decision on the general way of doing something. *'People voted for the Labour Party because they liked their policies.'*

9 False. A referendum is a vote where all the people of a country are asked to vote on a single question. *'We want a referendum on the issue of European Monetary Union.'*

10 False. An election is the process of choosing by voting. (The verb is *elect*.)

In Britain, a *general election* (in which all voters can vote for a government) is held every five years. When a Member of Parliament dies or retires, there is a *by-election* to choose a new MP.

Other words and expressions which you might find useful include:

- vote/elect/revolution/scandal/stand for – run for Parliament/seat/marginal seat/chamber/Vice-President/mayor/ambassador/embassy/party/representative/proportional representation/bureaucracy/bureaucrat

The three largest political parties in Britain are the *Labour Party*, the *Conservative Party* and the *Liberal Democrats*.

Page 122: The environment answers

Task 1

1. F (The opposite of *battery farming* is *free range* farming)   2. L   3. J (Some of these animals are called *protected species*, which means that it is illegal to kill them)   4. E   5. B   6. C   7. D   8. K
9. I   10. G   11. H   12. A (we can also use the word *hunting*, although there are some differences. *Poaching* means to *hunt illegally*)

Task 2

1. Green Belt   2. biodegradable packaging   3. greenhouse   4. rain forest   5. erosion
6. recycle   7. organic   8. genetically modified (we can also use the abbreviation *GM*)
9. unleaded petrol   10. Acid rain   11. ecosystem   12. emissions/fossil fuels
13. contaminated (we can also use the word *polluted*)   14. environmentalists   15. Global warming

Friends of the Earth and *Greenpeace* are two organisations which campaign to protect the environment. A third organisation, the *World Wide Fund for Nature* (*WWF*), protects endangered species of animals and plants and their habitats. They are also involved in projects to control pollution.

Task 3

1. fossil fuels   2. acid rain   3. greenhouse   4. global warming   5. rain forest
6. contaminated   7. emissions/gases   8. Poaching   9. endangered species   10. ecosystem
11. recycle   12. biodegradable   13. genetically modified   14. organic   15. unleaded petrol
16. environmentalists   17. conservation programmes   18. battery farming   19. Green Belts
Other words and expressions which you might find useful include:

- degradation/legislation/overfishing/greenhouse effect/ozone layer/destruction/waste disposal/overpopulation/bottle bank/carbon dioxide/climactic change/sea level/re-use/energy efficiency/radioactive waste/toxic waste/CFC gases

(For more information, *see* Collin PH and Greasby L (eds) (2001) *Dictionary of Ecology and Environment* (4e), published by Peter Collin Publishing)

Page 125: Healthcare answers

Task 1

1. D   2. G (a combination of 1 and 2 is called *rheumatoid arthritis*)   3. C   4. A   5. J
6. B   7. E   8. K   9. F (we can also say that their bodies *lack resistance to* illnesses)
10. H   (The *National Health Service* is a system of free doctors, nurses, hospitals and clinics run by the government in Britain. Many people in Britain prefer *private healthcare* because this is generally considered to be more efficient)
11. I

Task 2

1. therapeutic (the noun is *therapy*. A person who provides a therapeutic service is called a *therapist*)   2. a diet (this refers to the food we eat. If you go *on a diet*, you eat less in order to lose weight)   3. conventional medicine
4. traditional medicines   5. holistic medicine (an example of this is *aromatherapy*)   6. consultant
7. surgeon (*surgery* is the treatment of disease which requires an operation to cut into or remove part of the body. Do not confuse this with *a surgery*, which is a room where a normal doctor, sometimes called a *family doctor* or *general practitioner* – a *GP* – sees their patients)   8. protein   9. vitamins   10. minerals   11. active (the opposite of this is *sedentary* – see Task 1)   12. welfare state (other features of a welfare state include providing citizens with adequate housing, education and public transport)

Task 3

1. welfare state   2/3. cutbacks/underfunding (in either order)   4. conventional medicine   5. traditional medicine   6. arthritis   7. consultant (we can also use the word *specialist*)   8. surgery
9. therapeutic   10. stress-related   11. holistic medicine   12. diet   13/14. vitamins/minerals (in either order)   15. active   16. sedentary   17. cancer

Other words and expressions which you might find useful include:

* prescription/mental health/physical health/blood system/National Insurance/research/the World Health Organisation (the WHO)/blood pressure/cure/curable/incurable/remedy/prevention/operating theatre

(For more information, *see* Collin PH (2000) *Dictionary of Medicine* (3e), published by Peter Collin Publishing)

Page 128: Travel answers

Task 1

1. False. A travel agency (we sometimes use the expression *travel agent*) is a shop where you go to buy a holiday or a ticket. A tour operator is the company which sells the holiday to you *via* the travel agent.
2. True.
3. True.
4. False. They get *on* an aeroplane or ship.
5. False. They get *off* an aeroplane or ship.
6. True.
7. True.
8. True. (We can also use the word *backpacker*, describing somebody who carries a rucksack.)
9. True.
10. False. Eco-tourism is supposed to be tourism that *helps* the environment.

11. False. They are all slightly different. Use a dictionary to check these differences.
12. False. It depends from which country you come and where you are going. Citizens of the EU, for example, do not need visas if they are flying to another EU country.
13. False. It is a *short-haul* flight.
14. False. It is cheaper. (We can also use the expression *tourist class* instead of *economy class*.)
15. True. But see 12 above.

Task 2

1. refugees   2. internally displaced   3. emigration   4. immigration   5. culture shock
6. expatriates (often shortened to *expats*)   7. UNHCR (the United Nations High Commission for Refugees)
8. deported   9. persona non grata (a Latin expression which describes a foreign person, usually a diplomat, who is not acceptable to a government)   10. economic migrants   11. repatriated/deported

Task 3

1. travel agency   2. package tour   3. independent travellers   4. visas   5. check in
6. economy class   7. disembark   8. mass tourism   9. all-inclusive   10. eco-tourism
11. refugees   12. internally displaced   13. economic migrants   14. expatriates   15. culture shock
16. immigration   17. persona non grata   18. deported   19. checking in   20. excursion
Other words and expressions which you might find useful include:

• acclimatise/embassy/alien/illegal alien/check out/insurance/first class/cruise/sightseeing holiday/safari/adventure holiday/ skiing holiday/hotel/guest house/full-board/half-board/bed and breakfast/self-catering/suitcase/overnight bag

Page 130: Crime and the law answers

Task 1

1. judge   2. jury   3. witness   4. defendant   5. victim   6. solicitor (an *attorney* in the USA)
7. offender   8. barrister   9. law-abiding

Task 2

• Part 1: (In order) A, F, D, B, C, E
• Part 2: (In order) A, E, F, C, B, D
• Part 3: (In order) A, D, F, C, E (we can also use the expression *state punishment*), B

Task 3

1. committed   2. arrested/charged   3. court   4. pleaded   5. guilty   6. sentenced
7. misdeeds   8. law-abiding/innocent   9. retribution   10. rehabilitate/reform   11. reform
12. released   13. deterrent   14. parole   15. victim   16. offender   17. community service
18. fine   19/20. corporal punishment/capital punishment (in either order)   21/22. judges/barristers/solicitors/ juries (any of these in any order)
Other words and expressions which you might find useful include:

• lawyer/accuse/pass a verdict/send to prison/convict (noun + verb)/conviction/statement/wrongdoer/punish/punishment/ revenge/admit/deny

- *Different types of crime and criminal:* burglary – burglar/robbery – robber/shoplifting – shoplifter/vandalism – vandal/rape – rapist/hooliganism – hooligan/murder – murderer/hijack – hijacker/
- forgery – forger/espionage – spy/piracy – pirate/terrorism – terrorist etc . . .

(For more information, *see* Collin PH (2000) *Dictionary of Law* (3e), published by Peter Collin Publishing)

Page 132: Social tensions answers

Task 1

A. 10   B. 7   C. 1   D. 5   E. 3   F. 6   G. 8   H. 9   I. 2   J. 4

Task 2

ethnic cleansing – racial purging   prejudice – discrimination   civil rights – human rights   harassment – intimidation   rebel – non-conformist (the opposite of this is a *conformist*)   picket line – blackleg   poverty-stricken – destitute   refugee – displaced person   outcast – reject

Task 3

1. extremists   2. ethnic cleansing/genocide   3. Dissidents/Refugees   4. (political) asylum
5. illegal aliens   6. (institutional) racism   7. harassment/intimidation   8. Civil rights/Human rights   9. human rights/civil rights   10. Rebels   11. power struggle   12. homeless
13. poverty   14. squatters   15/16. discrimination/exploitation (in either order)   17. blacklegs
18. riots/unrest
   Other words and expressions which you might find useful include:

- discrimination/sectarian/multi-racial/multi-cultural/unorthodox/disparate/itinerant/community

Page 134: Science and technology answers

Task 1

1. research   2. development   3. innovations   4. react   5. invented
6. discovered   7. analysed   8. combined   9. a technophobe   10. a technophile
11. safeguards   12. an experiment   13. genetic engineering   14. molecular biology
15. cybernetics   16. nuclear engineering   17. breakthrough   18. life expectancy

Task 2

1. base unit/disk drive   2. hardware   3. load   4. software   5. monitor
6. printer   7. keyboard   8. mouse   9. scanner   10. log on   11. the Internet
12. web site   13. download   14. e-mail   15. crashed

Task 3

1. discovered   2. life expectancy   3. innovations   4. breakthrough   5. invented
6. Internet (we can also use the expression *world wide web*)   7. e-mail   8. research
9. technophiles   10. technophobes   11. cybernetics   12. nuclear engineering
13. safeguards   14. genetic engineering   15. analysed   16. experiment
    Other words and expressions which you might find useful include:

* information technology/bioclimatology/geopolitics/chemistry/physics/cryogenics + other specialised scientific or technological fields

Page 137: Food and diet answers

Task 1

1. calories   2. protein   3. carbohydrate   4. fat   5. fibre (we can also use the word
roughage)   6. cholesterol   7. vitamin   8. mineral (we often talk about the vitamin or mineral *content* of
a food)   9. overweight (if somebody is very overweight, we can say they are *obese*)
10. malnourished   11. nutrition (we often talk about the *nutritional value* of a food. The adjective is *nutritious*. A
person who specialises in the study of nutrition and advises on diets is called a *nutritionist*)

> Note: Fats in food come under four categories: saturated fat (which contains the largest amount of hydrogen possible);
> unsaturated fat; polyunsaturated fat (which is less likely to be converted into cholesterol in the body); and monounsaturated fat.

Task 2

1. H   2. C   3. A   4. I   5. D   6. E   7. B   8. F   9. J   10. G

Task 3

1. fast food   2/3. minerals/vitamins (in either order)   4/5. fat/carbohydrates (in either order)
6. malnutrition (the adjective is *malnourished*)   7. scarcity   8. harvest   9. balanced diet
10. fibre   11. fat/cholesterol   12. calories   13. Genetically modified   14. organic
15/16. salmonella/listeria (in either order)   17. food poisoning
    Other words and expressions which you might find useful include:

* consume/consumption/underweight/eating disorder/anorexia/anorexic/bulimia/bulimic/vegetarian/vegan/health foods

Page 140: Children and the family answers

Task 1

1. nuclear   2. extended   3. single-parent   4. bring up (we can also use the words *raise* or *rear*)
5. upbringing   6. divorced   7. childcare   8. adolescence (the noun is *adolescent*)

9. formative   10. birth rate   11. dependant (the adjective is *dependent*)   12. juvenile delinquency (in Britain, a juvenile is anybody below the age of 18, which is the age at which somebody becomes legally responsible for their own actions)

Task 2

1. H (*authoritarian* can be a noun and an adjective)   2. C   3. G   4. K   5. A   6. D
7. J (we can also use the expression *over-caring*)   8. B   9. E   10. F   11. I   12. L

Task 3

1. formative   2. divorced   3. brought up   4. foster family (a child who is raised by a foster family is called a *foster child*. The verb is *to foster*)   5. authoritarian   6. upbringing   7. running wild
8. adolescence   9. juvenile delinquency   10. responsible   11. siblings   12. well-adjusted
13. lenient   14. over-protective   15. nuclear   16. single-parent   17. dependants
18. extended

Other words and expressions which you might find useful include:

• abuse/rebelliousness/relationship/supervision/minor/relatives/nurture/kin/family life/split up/broken home/divorce rate

Page 142: On the road answers

Task 1

1. A   2. B   3. B   4. A   5. A   6. B   7. A   8. A   9. A   10. A
11. A   12. A

Task 2

1. D   2. H   3. F   4. A   5. J   6. G   7. C   8. I   9. E   10. B

Note:
Most large towns and cities in Britain have 'Park and Ride' schemes. These are large car parks outside city centres where drivers can park their car, usually for free. They can then take a bus into the city centre.
   Distances and speed limits in Britain are in miles or miles per hour (1 mile = 1.6 kilometres). The maximum speed limit in Britain is 60 mph on single-lane roads outside towns, or 70 mph on dual-carriageways or motorways. In most towns and cities, the maximum speed limit is usually 20 or 30 mph. Drivers who are caught speeding can face penalties ranging from a fine to imprisonment, depending on how fast they are driving and where. They can also have their driving licence suspended.
   Drink driving is considered a very serious offence. Offenders automatically have their driving licence suspended for at least a year, will normally receive a fine and may go to prison.

Task 3

1/2. injuries/fatalities (in either order)   3. speeding   4. drink-driving   5. pedestrians
6. pedestrian   crossings   7. Highway Code   8/9. congestion/pollution (in either order)
10. black spot   11. transport strategy   12. Traffic calming   13. Park and Ride
14. traffic-free zone   15. cycle lanes   16. subsidised   17. fines   18. dominate

Other words and expressions which you might find useful include:

* Objects in the street: zebra crossing/pelican crossing/traffic island/pavement/bollard/kerb/junction/crossroads/traffic cones
* Motorway/highway/carriageway/slip road/hard shoulder/central reservation/overtake/cut in/swerve/skid/brake/accelerate/lorry/articulated lorry/van/diesel

Page 145: The arts answers

Task 1

1. a ballet
2. a play
3. a biography (if somebody writes a book about themselves, we call it an *autobiography*)
4. a sculpture
5. a portrait
6. an opera
7. a concert
8. a novel
9. poetry
10. a still life

Task 2

1. C
2. A
3. B
4. A
5. C
6. B (we can also use the word *grant*)
7. C
8. C (we can also use the word *writers*)
9. B (*impressionism* is the name we give to this genre of painting)
10. A

Task 3

1. ballet
2. performance
3. reviews
4. exhibition
5. Gallery
6. portraits
7. still life
8. subsidy
9. novelist
10. works/novels
11. published
12. biography
13. concert
14. opera
15. sculpture

Other words and expressions which you might find useful include:

* a musical/produce/production/exhibit/artist/actor/author/sculptor/collection/pop art

Page 148: Town and country answers

Task 1

1. N
2. M
3. G
4. A
5. I
6. B
7. C
8. F
9. H
10. E
11. K
12. D
13. L
(we can also say *CBD*)
14. J

Task 2

1. H
2. B
3. G
4. F
5. A
6. C
7. E
8. D

Task 3

1. metropolis
2. cosmopolitan
3. urban
4. amenities
5. cultural events
6. infrastructure
7. commuters
8. Central Business District
9. rush hour/peak periods
10. congestion
11. pollution
12. cost of living
13. building sites
14. population explosion
15. drug abuse
16. inner-city
17. rural
18. prospects
19. productive land/cultivation/arable land
20. urban sprawl
21. environment

Other words and expressions which you might find useful include:

• suburbs/facilities/employment/unemployment/resident/residential/outskirts/property prices/development

Page 151: Architecture answers

Task 1

• Building materials: timber/stone/steel/glass/concrete/reinforced concrete
• Aesthetic perception: well-designed/an eyesore/elegant/ugly/controversial/pleasing geometric forms
• Types of building: skyscraper/low-rise apartments/high-rise apartments (in Britain, the word *flat* is usually used instead of *apartment*)/multi-storey car park
• Architectural style: modernist/post-modern/standardised/traditional/international style/art deco (high-tech could also be included here)
• Parts of a building: porch/façade/walls/foundations
• Features: practical/functional/high-tech/energy-efficient

Task 2

1. B   2. A   3. C   4. C   5. A   6. A   7. C   8. C   9. A   10. A

Task 3

1. planning   2. preservation   3. renovate   4. architects   5. glass   6. façade
7. foundations   8. social   9. derelict   10. estate   11. an eyesore   12. traditional
13. slums   14. high-rise/low-rise   15. energy-efficient

Other words and expressions which you might find useful include:

• Other types of building: detached house/semi-detached house/terraced house/mansion/cottage/manor house/bungalow/maisonette/castle/palace/shopping centre (in the USA – shopping *mall*)
• Other parts of a building: roof/ground floor (in the USA = first floor)/first floor (in the USA = second floor)/basement (cellar)/attic/staircase
• Verbs: construct/design/plan/modernise
• Others: standardised/prefabricated/development/mass-produced/low-cost

Page 154: Men and women answers

Task 1

• These words and expressions generally have **positive** connotations: astute   multi-faceted   egalitarian   equality
• These words and expressions generally have **negative** connotations: power struggle   ruthless   weaker sex (a derogatory, slightly old-fashioned expression referring to women)   male chauvinist (the expression *male chauvinist pig* can also be used, although it is considered insulting)   sex objects   male-dominated   militant feminists (although some women would argue that this has positive connotations)

Task 2

1. household management (we also use the expressions *domestic chores* or *housework*)   2. Sex Discrimination Act (a British law which states that men and women should be treated equally, with equal pay, terms and conditions for doing the same job etc)   3. male counterparts   4. child rearing   5. role division (we sometimes write *role* as *rôle*)   6. breadwinner (we can also use the expression *financial provider*)   7. social convention   8. gender roles   9. stereotypes   10. battle of the sexes

Task 3

1. egalitarian   2. equality   3. breadwinner   4. weaker sex   5. stereotypes   6. gender roles   7. male-dominated   8. ruthless   9. astute   10. multi-faceted   11. Sex Discrimination Act   12. male chauvinist   13. role division   14. child rearing   15. household management   16. Social convention   17. militant feminists   18. sex objects   19. power struggle/battle of the sexes   20. male counterparts   21. battle of the sexes/power struggle
  Other words and expressions which you might find useful include:

- discriminate/second class citizens/unisex/sexist/exploitation/cohabit/masculine – feminine qualities/modern man (a relatively new expression describing a man who believes in total equality between men and women and is happy to do tasks previously considered only suitable for a woman)

Page 157: Geography answers

Task 1

1	tree	copse	wood	forest	(*beach* does not belong here)
2	footpath	track	lane	road	(*peak* does not belong here)
3	hillock	hill	mountain	mountain range	(*shore* does not belong here)
4	hollow	gorge	valley	plain	(*waterfall* does not belong here)
5	inlet	cove	bay	gulf	(*ridge* does not belong here)
6	brook	stream	river	estuary	(*cliff* does not belong here)
7	city	county	country	continent	(*tributary* does not belong here)
8	puddle	pond	lake	sea	ocean	(*cape* does not belong here)

Task 2

- *Geographical features associated with water and the sea:* coast   peninsula   shore   beach   cape   source   coastline   tributary   waterfall   mouth   cliff
- *Geographical features associated with land, hills and mountains:* mountainous   ridge   cliff   summit   glacier   plateau   peak   highlands
- *Words associated with agriculture and rural land:* depopulation   fertile   under-developed   vegetation   irrigation
- *Words associated with towns and cities:* urban sprawl   densely populated   industrialised   conurbation   overcrowding

Task 3

1. densely populated   2. industrialised   3. urban sprawl   4. city   5. irrigation   6. source
7. peaks   8. mountain range   9. depopulation   10. Valley   11. waterfalls   12. streams
13. lane   14. track   15. Ocean   16. cape/peninsula   17. hills   18. plain   19. delta
20. fertile   21. shore/beach   22. country
   Other words and expressions which you might find useful include:

* lowlands/mountainous/hilly/flat/climate/diverse

Page 160: Business and industry answers

Task 1

1. demand for   2. loss   3. net   4. lending   5. credit   6. retail   7. private
8. State-owned industries   9. Unskilled labourers   10. take on (we can also use the word *employ*)
11. White-collar   12. exports   13. bust/recession   14. employees/workers/staff
15. expenditure   16. shop floor

Task 2

1. F   2. L   3. O   4. H   5. M   6. C (GNP = Gross National Product. Compare this with
GDP – Gross Domestic Product)   7. A   8. E   9. B   10. G   11. K   12. J
13. D   14. P   15. Q (VAT = Value Added Tax)   16. I   17. N

Task 3

1. Interest   2. borrowing   3. lay off   4. unemployment   5. Inflation   6. exports
7. secondary industries   8. Blue-collar/White-collar   9. state-owned/nationalised   10. salaries
11. management   12. public   13. Demand   14. supply   15. revenue/income
16. nationalised   17. deficit   18. automation
   See Module 36: Work and Module 37: Money and finance for other words and expressions which you might find useful.
   (For more information, *see* Collin PH (2004) *Dictionary of Business* (4e), published by Peter Collin Publishing)

Page 163: Global problems answers

Task 1

1. B   2. A   3. B   4. C   5. A   6. C   7. A   8. B   9. A
10. C   11. B   12. B   13. A   14. B   15. A

Note: A hurricane is the name we give to a tropical storm with strong winds and rain in the Caribbean or Eastern Pacific. In the Far East it is called a *typhoon*. In the Indian Ocean it is called a *cyclone*.

Task 2

1. spread   2. spread/swept   3. erupted   4. shook   5. broke out   6. casualties
7. survivors/casualties   8. Refugees/Survivors   9. suffering   10. relief
(These words do not belong anywhere: disaster/spouted/ran/flamed/wobbled)

Task 3

1. torrential   2. flood   3. epidemic   4. famine   5. relief   6. volcano
7. erupted   8. hurricane   9. devastation   10. typhoon   11. casualties   12. drought
13. civil war   14. Refugees/Survivors   15. swept/spread   16. accident   17. explosions
18. plague
Other words and expressions which you might find useful include:

* major (accident)/disease/illness/hardship/dead/wounded/injured/homeless/victim/aid convoy

See also Module 43: Social tensions.

Appendix: Registration with the General Medical Council (GMC)

Who needs to take IELTS

All overseas qualified doctors who apply for limited, provisional or full registration must satisfy the GMC that they have the necessary knowledge of English. They are accordingly required to obtain satisfactory scores in each of the four academic modules (speaking, listening, writing and reading) of the IELTS test. The only exceptions, under European law, are:

- Nationals of member states of the European Economic Area (EEA) other than the UK.

- Swiss nationals who since 1 June 2002 benefit under European law.

- UK nationals who have exercised, or are exercising, their European Community (EC) rights of free movement within the EEA. Generally speaking, exercising EC rights of free movement in this context means that the person must have worked as a doctor in another EEA member state and be returning to the UK to take up employment.

- UK nationals and non-EEA nationals who are married to EEA nationals who are exercising, or have exercised, their EC rights of free movement within the EEA. Generally speaking, exercising EC rights of free movement in this context means that the spouse must be coming to the UK to take up employment.

The GMC is not able to give detailed guidance on what a person needs to do in order to exercise EC rights of free movement as this is a legal concept. Any doctor who wishes to be advised about this should contact a lawyer or a citizens advice bureau (CAB).

It is unlawful for the GMC to impose a test of linguistic competence upon EEA nationals of an EEA member state other than the UK, or upon others with enforceable EC rights, at the point of registration. Responsibility for ensuring that such doctors' proficiency in written and spoken English is sufficient for the purpose of their employment is a matter for the employing authority.

How to apply

IELTS is administered jointly by the British Council and IDP Education Australia and is run in over 100 countries. You can obtain further information from the IELT's website at www.ielts.org or from:

British Council National Advice Centre
Bridgewater House
58 Whitworth Street
Manchester M1 6BB
Telephone: 0161 957 7218
Fax: 0161 957 7029
Email: general.enquiries@britishcouncil.org
www.britishcouncil.org/health

What scores are required?

The scores required vary depending on whether you take the PLAB test or not. This is because doctors who take the PLAB test have an additional assessment of their communication skills in Part 2 of the PLAB test.

If you are not taking the PLAB test you need to obtain a minimum score of 7.0 in each of the 4 academic modules (speaking, listening, writing and reading).

If you are planning to take the PLAB test you must obtain an overall score of 7.0 with minimum scores of 7.0 in speaking and 6.0 in reading, writing and listening.

All doctors must obtain the minimum scores required in one sitting of the IELTS test.

You should be aware that the GMC is currently reviewing its experience of the IELTS test as a method for testing language skills. It is likely that this work will also consider whether a lower score for those taking the PLAB test continues to be justified.

How long is the IELTS report form valid for?

If your pass in the IELTS test is more than two years old at whichever is the earlier of the date your registration is granted or (where appropriate) the date you passed Part 1 of the PLAB test, you will need to provide proof that you have maintained your English language skills since you passed the IELTS tests. The ways in which you can do this include:

• Sending proof to the GMC that you have undertaken a postgraduate course of study (where the language of instruction and examination was in English) within the last two years and since you took your IELTS test. You will also need to send your original IELTS certificate showing that you acquired the required scores.

or

- Sending a reference to the GMC completed by a UK employer or your tutor or lecturer on a postgraduate course of study within the last two years since you took your IELTS test. You will also need to send the GMC your original IELTS certificate showing that you acquired the required scores.

or

- Sending proof to the GMC that you have taken the IELTS test again and attained the required scores.

The GMC will consider whether you will be exempt from retaking the IELTS test.

Contacting us

Email: registrationhelp@gmc-uk.org
Phone: (+44) (0)20 7915 3630
Fax: (+44) (0)20 7915 3532
Write: Registration Services
General Medical Council
178 Great Portland Street
London W1W 5JE

Vocabulary record sheet

Use this sheet to develop your own bank of useful words and expressions.

Word or expression	Definition	Sample sentence(s)